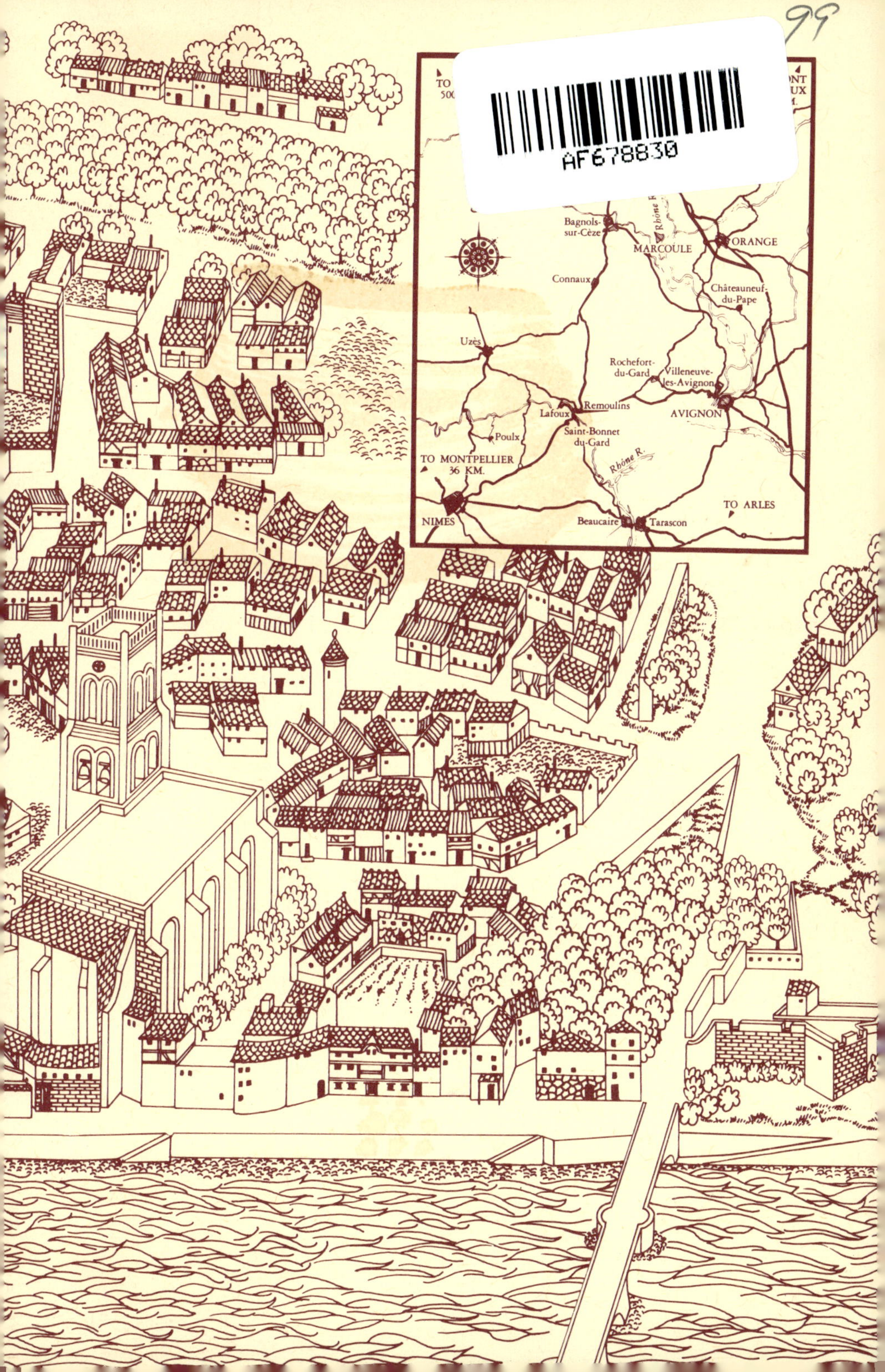
Bagnols-
sur-Cèze
MARCOULE
ORANGE
Connaux
Châteauneuf-
du-Pape
Uzès
Rochefort-
du-Gard
Villeneuve-
les-Avignon
Remoulins
Lafoux
AVIGNON
Saint-Bonnet
du-Gard
Poulx
TO MONTPELLIER
36 KM.
Rhône R.
NIMES
Beaucaire
Tarascon
TO ARLES

BY JOHN G. FULLER

The Day of St. Anthony's Fire

The Interrupted Journey

Incident at Exeter

The Money Changers

The Gentlemen Conspirators

Games for Insomniacs

THE DAY OF ST. ANTHONY'S FIRE

THE DAY OF ST. ANTHONY'S FIRE

John G. Fuller

The Macmillan Company, *New York*

Library of Congress Catalog Card Number 68-23632

First Printing

The Macmillan Company, New York
Collier-Macmillan Canada Ltd., Toronto, Ontario

Printed in the United States of America

THE DAY OF ST. ANTHONY'S FIRE

ONE

THE STATUE of the Virgin, tall as three men, could hardly be seen through the rain that whipped the countryside that May morning in 1951. Father Jurand, squeezing out of a car in the courtyard of the château of Notre Dame de la Bache, had less thought then of the Virgin and the high tower she stood on than he did of arriving at the château reasonably dry and presentable. Bending against the wind, he hurried toward the stone steps gathering his black robes, already soaked, around his legs. At that moment he heard the sound above the wind, a crushing, sickening sound from the top of the *colline,* unmistakably from the tower that dominated the château from some hundred and fifty yards away. Startled, he strained to look through the rain, to the tower, to the statue six stories above the ground. The Virgin was there still, her head tilted down in an attitude of grace, as she had been since 1848. But Father Jurand could tell, even from the distance, that instead of her arms being extended in the manner of the Virgin *de la médaille miraculeuse,* only the right arm was visible. All that remained of the left was a shattered stump. Quickly, he wiped the rain from his eyes, and entered the doors of the château to bring the news to *les Frères des Écoles Chrétiennes*. His mission had changed from that of a casual visitor to that of a courier of unwelcome news. The brothers of Notre Dame de la Bache would hardly embrace the event with enthusiasm.

Tragedy had come to the stone Madonna before, not more than twelve years ago. On the eve of the Second World War in 1939, a bolt of lightning had shattered the statue with such force that it plunged to the hilltop sixty feet below the tower, in fragments. There were some in the village nearby at that time who said that this bitter adversity preordained a coming catastrophe. They had the grim satisfaction of seeing their forecast proved when the war struck France with all its fury only days afterward.

Now, twelve years later, in 1951, the villagers would again look up to the high hill towering above the plains of the Rhône Valley to see the statue of the beloved Virgin lacking the left arm and without the symmetry they had come to take as a matter of course.

By the time the sun returned, the tragedy of the Virgin—Notre Dame de la Bache—would be known in the villages and throughout the countryside. From almost any vineyard on the plain, from the nearby villages spread along the Rhône, the statue dominates the scene. In turn, from her imposing pedestal, the Virgin looks down with a granite serenity on a tapestry of rich and fertile vineyards, neatly carpeting the plain, toward the Rhône, toward the village of Pont-Saint-Esprit just three kilometers away. In the distance, across the Rhône, the massive peak of Mont Ventoux looms in full view, and beyond it in the great distance, the Alps and Italy. To the south, the Rhône Valley sweeps down past Bagnols-sur-Cèze, toward Avignon, Beaucaire, Nîmes, and Arles, where there is history under every stone. All along the Rhône Valley, the ruins of castles cling like stalagmites to the crusty peaks on either side of the river, most of their ramparts smashed by Richelieu's fist when the nobles of the Midi tried their half-hearted rebellion after the ruthless and insane Wars of Religion.

In spite of her lost arm, the Virgin statue surveyed a peaceful, if not a ravishing scene in that spring of 1951. Only the Rhône was turbulent, but that would be expected of a river which had led many strong *mariniers* from Vernaison or Condrieu to pray as much as they navigated. The chapels on and under the bridges of

Pont-Saint-Esprit and Avignon testify to that. Here the mariners would pray that their skill, their navigation secrets, handed down for generations, would take them past the hazards that had wrecked so many of their boats and sent countless treasures down to the bottom of the then-untamable Rhône.

The charm, the loveliness, the strange and indescribable luminosity of Provence and Languedoc—for Pont-Saint-Esprit sits on the dividing line between the two—has been praised lyrically by the troubadours, Stendhal, Dante, Petrarch, Mistral, Daudet, and others over the centuries. Pont-Saint-Esprit has been called by Frédéric Mistral "*la porte du Midi*"—the great moment in geography when the north of France dissolves into the romance and legend of the Midi, leaving the grayness of the north behind in favor of lavender, thyme, perfume, and the twisted trunks of olive trees. At Pont-Saint-Esprit also, the ranges of the Massif Central begin to give way to the more gentle Cévennes, and the tunnels of shade provided by the plane trees in the village are said to be enough to combat the broiling sun of the long summer months. "*C'est la porte sainte, la porte triomphale de la terre d'amour*," wrote Mistral of Pont-Saint-Esprit, forgetting in his enthusiasm the more bloody struggles of history played in this theater.

From her pedestal near the Rhône, the Virgin statue, whole or wounded, looks out on both the exuberant view reflected by Mistral and the ghost images of the sanguine combats of the past. Not far away the first big battle between the Romans and the Celts took place. Part of Hannibal's army plundered through the region on its way to Rome in 218 B.C., and the army of Bituit crossed the Rhône on a bridge of boats at the place where Pont-Saint-Esprit stands today.

The Middle Ages brought no rest from turbulence. Ten thousand Saracens were finally slaughtered nearby by Charles Martel in the ninth century. At that time, it was known as Saint-Saturnin-du-Port, and by 1164 the port was able to enjoy the spate of prosperity that lasted until Raymond the Seventh sacked the town in 1239.

By the beginning of the fourteenth century, the town was walled and fortified, and the bridge—many thought it was a religious miracle—was built across half a mile of untamed Rhône, with twenty-two arches. The towers on each end held a garrison of three hundred men, and from that moment on, no military operation would be carried out in the Rhône Valley that failed to involve Saint Saturnin. This was hardly a blessing, since the town went through a nightmare occupation by the *routiers,* involving the usual consequences of rape, murder, and pillage.

In May of 1951, after the storm that ripped the arm from the Virgin statue, the town and the valley bathed in the utter loveliness of the Midi springtime. The trim and manicured vines, born in Roman times and neighbors to the courtly Châteauneuf-du-Pape vineyards, the cypress trees, the myrtle, the peach blossoms, the lavender, could wipe out the memory of all the great historic hardship—and even the misfortune that had struck the Madonna.

During the days that followed, the townspeople and *les cultivateurs* would look up to the statue from great distances with regret. But there was work to do in the vineyards, and the merchants of Pont-Saint-Esprit were beginning to feel the growing pains brought on by the construction of the Donzère-Mondragon dam and power plants, which with the Centre d'Energie Atomique some ten kilometers below, would begin to change the medieval face of the countryside for miles around.

But some of the faithful could not forget the incident of the Virgin statue so quickly, even as the workmen began to repair it. They thought of the last time the storm had wrecked her stateliness, when the tragedy of the Second World War had followed so brusquely. Could the new distress of the statue be another omen that a tragedy was about to strike? Many talked about it in the market place the following Saturday morning, where by habit and tradition the stalls are set up each week under the plane trees along the Boulevard Gambetta and Boulevard Carnot. At the weekly market a bewildering variety of wares is displayed. Here the villagers buy trinkets, haberdashery, geraniums and begonias, hardware, fruits, and vegetables, spices and poultry—and even tractors. The market is the focal event of the week at Pont-Saint-Esprit, as it is all throughout Provence and Languedoc. It creates a scene of monumental gossip sessions embracing the latest scandal, jokes, and family news. At these moments the town becomes a giant, interrelated, and animated family, before the people return with overloaded baskets to the narrow, twisted streets of the ancient town, where even a *deux-chevaux* Citröen must brush the skirts of a passerby before it can get through the village.

On one of these streets—the rue des Quatre Coins—lived Mlle. Francine Rabassa, who, returning from the market that morning, pondered over the talk of the broken arm of the Madonna. She was religious, a good Catholic, but certainly not fanatic or superstitious. She did not believe in omens, or live by them. The suggestion, however, planted in her mind by the market gossip, continued to plague her for several days. She worked during the week on the Boulevard Gambetta at the combined home and office of M. and Mme. Eynard, a young husband and wife who had brought skilled and modern dentistry to the town, which was desperately in need of it.

"You know," she said one morning to Madame Eynard, who helped her husband in his practice only occasionally during this time because of their small daughter and a child she was carrying, "I do not like to think that I am superstitious. But this story of the arm falling off the statue of the Madonna keeps going through my mind."

"Why does it bother you so much?" Mme. Eynard asked.

"They say in the village that it is an omen," Francine said. "A very bad omen."

"I wouldn't pay much attention to that," Mme. Eynard said. "People are always going around trying to create ugly omens out of everything." Madame Eynard was a pragmatist, knowledgeable in the ways of the outside modern world. She was kind and sympathetic and well loved throughout the village, both as a dentist and as a person.

"The rumors are so *persistent,*" Francine continued. "Some even say that they *knew* the arm was going to fall off—before it happened."

Mme. Eynard laughed. "Some people claim to know everything before it happens. I usually find we don't have to pay much attention to them."

"The last time it happened," Francine said, "was on the eve of the Second World War. And that came about. Especially in this town." She was referring to the occupation by the Waffen SS, when the Nazis converted the ancient underground Citadel on the banks of the Rhône to interrogate and slaughter over four thousand members of the Resistance from all around the region. They would, conveniently, dump the bodies in the Rhône. This and the bombardment by the Allies on August 15, 1944, had left fresh scars on the town to add to those left by the violence of the Middle Ages.

"We have had much tragedy here," Mme. Eynard said. As an amateur historian she knew this well. She was later to plan a campaign to restore as historic monuments the Citadel and the unique Église Collégiale du Plan, the 1319 cathedral deep underground beside the Citadel, with its sculptured doorway built by Louis XI. "But perhaps now we'll be able to live in peace and help our town grow well again."

"Perhaps," said Francine. "I do hope so. We have had enough trouble."

"We have," said Madame Eynard. "Enough to think that maybe we'll deserve better times."

"Well," said Francine. "I'm going to forget about it. I just wanted to get it off my mind."

She did forget, and so did Madame Eynard. The mistral—the wind, not the poet—stopped its cruel whiplashing of the Valley for the summer months. The courtyards in the bent streets blossomed with roses and wisteria, and the romantic aura of Daudet's Provence took over the spirits of the people. The Ardèche and Rhône rivers gave over their trout and shad to the fisherman, the Ardèche also offering clear and sparkling refreshment to the swimmers of the town. For the more adventurous, the Mediterranean lay only two hours away. By the time August arrived, the hunters, intent on rabbit and thrush, were wiping down the barrels of their shotguns in anticipation of the coming hunting season, as the townspeople prepared for the yearly fête, the high mark of the year each September.

It was during these joyous summer days of 1951, on July 18, that *wagon* number 7.382.682 of the Société National Chemin de Fer, the railroad better known as the S.N.C.F., left the station at Chauvigny, some three hundred miles to the northeast of Pont-Saint-Esprit. The freight car included in its load ten quintals of flour, a quintal being a sack weighing one hundred kilograms. This flour would find its way to the bakeries of Pont-Saint-Esprit several weeks later, by way of Bagnols-sur-Cèze, the distribution center for the region. It was the first of several loads of flour to leave Chauvigny that month, and although no one knew it at the time, this small and routine event would shatter the peace of the village of Pont-Saint-Esprit for years to come.

Bread in France is more than the staff of life, it is a way of life. It is said that when the *boulanger* closes his shop, the village is doomed forever. In the Midi, the occasional ghost villages perched on mountaintops mark the beginning of their ends by the quiet retreat of the baker, his family, and his household goods to the more acceptable commerce of the valley towns.

In every French village, in the gray, sullen morning, or the bright and bustling noon hour, or when night approaches, the townspeople file in and out of the bakery carrying the crusty-brown *flûtes, baguettes,* and *gros pains* under their arms, often like cordwood when the size of the family demands it. To buy wrapped bread—*pain de mie*—or any bread far in advance of the meal is offensive to the sensitivity of the French. Fresh bread, straight from the oven, is a ritual; the bakeshop a shrine.

The villages in the constellation surrounding Pont-Saint-Esprit are no exception. With the heady and sometimes quarrelsome Tavel wine of the region, or the bracing Côtes-du-Rhône from nearby, the bread is an ideal companion to the rich southern meals of the Midi.

South of Pont-Saint-Esprit by some twenty kilometers is the village of Connaux, a tiny maze of stone houses squeezed together in random pattern, the twisted streets designed, so they say, to break the power of the mistral as it sweeps down valley from the Massif Central and the Alps.

There are twenty-two telephones in Connaux, representing one doctor, the *cave coopérative* of the wine growers, an electrician-plumber, a notary, two garages, a mason, Le Mairie, or town hall, a woodworker, and in the year 1951, two *boulangerie-pâtisserie* shops, one belonging to Monsieur Monier, the other to Monsieur Griotti.

On August 5, 1951, M. Monier found himself working especially hard because of *la fête votive* in the village, a festival marked with as much enthusiasm as the *Fête du Premier de Sep-*

tembre, which was to take place in a few weeks in the streets of the neighboring Pont-Saint-Esprit.

But tempering his enjoyment of the festival, as M. Monier labored in his bakeshop, was the fact that he was having extreme difficulty working the batter for the bread in which he took so much pride. The problem seemed to lie in the flour shipped to him by the Union Meunière, the giant distribution organization of France that supplies flour to the bakers through its distributors at strategically located centers throughout the country. It is not a union in the labor sense of the word. As a state-supervised private monopoly, its responsibilities are well defined, and its distribution is patterned so that if one *département*—as the regional sections of France are called—is lacking in flour, another will provide what is necessary to keep the distribution on an even keel.

The flour that caused him so much trouble that night of August 5 came from a miller unknown to him, far to the north, and what distressed M. Monier so much was that it was grayish in color, somewhat sticky, with an oilish texture which gave no promise of creating the rich and tasty bread he liked to deliver to his clients. He was able to meet his quota that night by mixing the flour with that of another sack from the nearby Vaucluse. Although the batter still did not shape to his artisan requirements, the bread rose and baked to a crisp brown turn, and its flavor met the requirements of his discerning tongue. He fumed, as other bakers were doing, at the lack of freedom to choose the source of his flour, because of the rigid regulations imposed by the Union Meunière's control of the distribution. There was no choice, and the baker had to accept what he received. To reject a shipment of flour was tantamount to closing down the shop for several days in the hope it could be proved that his instinctual evaluation of the flour could stand up against the appraisal of the chemists assigned to check it.

That same night, in Connaux, the baker Griotti was having his own problems with the batter made from the flour of M. Maillet, who was the miller from the north supplying the region at that time. Like his *confrère,* M. Griotti found that he could work the dough only by mixing it with a flour from a neighboring region, and he barely managed to turn out his product for the heavy Monday morning trade through this device.

By Monday afternoon both M. Monier and M. Griotti began to receive visitors in their respective *boulangeries.* They were the regular customers of the day before, and their complaints were nearly identical: violent colic after eating the bread. By evening M. Griotti, his wife, and his six-year-old daughter were stricken, as well as the other members of his family in the household. They suffered not only from colic, but from diarrhea, and eruptions of a rash over the skin. M. Griotti went immediately to the café, the heart and center of every French village, where he discovered more of his clients who were ill, and learned also that several clients of M. Monier had registered the same complaints. He continued on quickly to his *confrère's* establishment, where both of them decided to set aside the suspect flour immediately, and lodge a strong protest with the Union Meunière.

They did, each of them writing to the organization's headquarters for the département du Gard in nearby Nîmes. They were morally supported by the secretary of the bakers' association of Gard, who happened to be in Connaux for the votive festival. By Wednesday, August 8, they were assured by the director of the Union Meunière in Nîmes that their complaints would be taken care of by M. Bousquet, the local distributor who operated out of Bagnols-sur-Cèze, halfway between Connaux and Pont-Saint-Esprit.

M. Jean Bousquet, since 1944 *le répartiteur des farines,* or distributor, in the area, was having more troubles than the Connaux *boulangers.* Practically every baker in the region who had received shipments of flour coming from the Maillet mill in the north was protesting vigorously about the quality. In the village of Saint-Génies-de-Comolas the local baker became so distressed he called the mayor of the town to his shop to show him the flour. The dough formed from it was greasy, slimy, and gray, and the mayor immediately forbade the baker to use it, lodging his own protest with M. Bousquet as well as with the *préfet* of the *département.* On August 9, M. Bousquet sat down to write in urgency to his superiors in the Union Meunière office at Nîmes:

"*Nous vous signalons à toutes fins utiles que presque tous les boulangers du centre de Bagnols se plaignant de la qualité des farines qui sont en provenance de M. Maillet,*" he wrote, pointing out sharply that nearly all his clients were grumbling about the flour coming from the one mill and that action needed to be taken.

While waiting for action from the flour monopoly, which seemed remarkably slow in arriving, M. Bousquet continued to dole out his supplies, rationing the flour of the Maillet mill with other stock from a different region. By contract the Union authorities must immediately take five samples of any flour, about which complaints are made, to be analyzed. No provisions in the cumbersome mechanics of distribution had been made about what the bakers should do in the interim. They in turn were not allowed to shut down without express permission. Further, the grain did not seem seriously defective. The problem seemed to be mainly a question of a temporary bread supply of slightly inferior quality. There seemed to be no threat of further illnesses, which had died off after the initial flurry in Connaux. One strange symptom did, however, continue. The family of M. Griotti discovered that they had difficulty getting to sleep, and this condition lasted for several days.

A further complication plagued the bakers of the area in that the lumbering distribution system made it impossible for them to refuse delivery of the flour, their only right being to notify the Union of any problems with the supplies.

After several telephone calls to the flour monopoly at Nîmes, M. Bousquet's patience began to wear thin, along with the nerves of his clients, who continued to protest to him. He wrote again to the Union Meunière on August 11, demanding immediate instructions. He received none. By August 13 a group of bakers from the towns around gathered in his office to threaten severe action if the Union did not respond to their complaints. At eleven o'clock that morning M. Bousquet called directly to the Union headquarters at Nîmes in the presence of the angry bakers. He was assured politely that someone would be around to gather the necessary samples. The bakers, temporarily mollified, went back to their shops to work with the material they had on hand. M. Bousquet, bristling under both the delays of the Union Meunière and the pressure from the bakers, faced frustration in any direction he looked. At the end of the unwelcome conference, he wrote again to headquarters, his anger bursting through the usual reserve he employed in his letters.

"*. . . en vous demandant à ce que* de toute urgence *des PRÉLÈVEMENTS D'ÉCHANTILLONS,*" he wrote, referring to the urgency of at least taking the samples of the flour, if nothing else. By Friday, August 17, his patience was obliterated as the mayor of Saint-Génies-de-Comolas arrived at his office to warn him that unless the Union Meunière took immediate action, the mayor would organize every town in the vicinity to demand action.

For the fourth time M. Bousquet sat down at his desk to write the Union, this time with the despair and exhaustion that can only come from dealing with the impossible phantom created by a giant, impersonal organization.

But even as he wrote the letter, the germination of one of the strangest, most inexplicable tragedies of modern medical history had already been set in motion, and nothing that M. Bousquet or the Union Meunière might now do could stop it. For that matter, nothing in known modern medical practice could combat it.

On the road north from Bagnols toward Pont-Saint-Esprit, over the crest of the last hill, the plains of the Rhône sprawl out in a magnificent vista, with the rust-red rooftops of the village marking the random, crooked lines of the streets and *allées* which defy geometry. While the ramparts are no longer surrounding the town, the demarcation lines are still visible, as if the turrets, with their pikemen and crossbowmen were still there in ghost image. Above the town the tower of the fifteenth-century Église Saint-Saturnin surveys the tile roofs with a placid acceptance of all the indignities history has brought to the village. In the bright morning sunlight of the Midi, the winding streets and oddly pitched roofs take on the aspect of the illustrations of a fairy-tale book. Over many streets and ways are ancient arches, with the *allées* snaking under them to become lost in the rest of the maze. A stranger in the center of the old town can lose his way in moments in the unpredictable turnings of the streets. For even a medium-sized American automobile, the ways are impassable.

Along the new concrete dikes of the Rhône banks the ancient houses show their backs to the river. At one time during the Middle Ages their windows were walled in to become part of the fortress against the marauding *routiers.*

The bridge at Pont-Saint-Esprit is the pride of both the town and history. Its more famous sister bridge, forty kilometers below at Avignon, has not stood the test of posterity as well. Only a fragment remains of the latter, under which they used to dance on the grassy island in the Rhône, rather than on the bridge itself, as the song suggests. At the second half of the thirteenth century *les frères pontifes* were invited by Pont-Saint-Esprit to duplicate their miraculous work at Avignon. In spite of the inspiration of the Holy Spirit, the new bridge took from 1265 to 1309 to complete.

Today the ancient stone arches of the bridge support the rumbling tracks and traffic of Route National 94, just as they did the wagons and carts of the Middle Ages. At the Pont-Saint-Esprit end of the bridge only the stately Maison du Roy, where twelve different kings of France were received, remains above ground to mark the entrance to the town.

Bending through the old village, from the place de la République to the place de l'Hôtel de Ville is the narrow street known as Grande Rue. Its width—barely enough to permit four people to pass—and its total lack of sidewalks belie its name. Yet it is an important street for both its merchants and its residents. It is, in a sense, the gravitational center of town, even if it does lack the all-important cafés that find more room for their sprawling outdoor tables under the plane trees of the Boulevards Gambetta and Carnot.

There are almost no phones on Grande Rue, even among the commercial establishments. Perhaps it is because the tight compression of the streets and the medieval houses make it possible to talk face-to-face across the window sills or from the doorways, and sooner or later everyone in the village is likely to find himself on the Grande Rue at one time or another during the week. There is on the street nearly all that human needs might demand: A *droguerie* for hardware, paints, tools, nails, glue, sandpaper, toothpaste, O'Cedar mops, shaving cream, and toilet needs; a *fleuriste* for the absolute necessity of pleasing the aesthetic taste of the French; a seed store, to supply the means to grow a villager's own flowers; a *boucherie-charcuterie,* where sausages and the best French cuts of meats may be had; a *pharmacie,* strictly for medicines of any type, whether they are prescribed or not—and without the soda fountain or extras; *électricité générale,* including wiring, lamp fixtures, television, radio, and light bulbs; *une boutique des vêtements*, with clothing for infants, and a *chemiserie* and *bonneterie* for adults; a *poissonnerie*, for fish and sea food, raw materials for the popular Provençal *bouillabaisse;* an *alimentation*, for foods and *vin courant;* and, of course, the *boulangerie* and *pâtisserie*, the most-frequented shops on any street.

In August of 1951 the most popular baker on the Grande Rue was Roche Briand. Powerful, tall, athletic, in his forties, he served his clients well, priding himself in the rich, golden loaves he stacked on end each day behind his counter, taking equal pride in the *brioches* and *croissants* he baked. He was known among the residents of Grande Rue to go out of his way to help a client who needed information in the more complex things of the outside world, such as tax information, insurance data, or minor legal problems, since Pont-Saint-Esprit did not have the luxury of a full-time lawyer, or *avocat*. Part of his time, as a matter of fact, was devoted to insurance work. For thirty years his bakery had served the town well, and many claimed his bread was the best in the region. Since 1925 he had been married to Marie Jeanne, and he had two daughters and two sons ranging from twenty-three to eleven. In September of 1939 he had joined *des troupes coloniales* in Marseilles, and spent thirteen months of his service in Syria.

During the time that M. Bousquet was doling out and rationing the questionable flour from the north, M. Briand and the other bakers of Pont-Saint-Esprit added their protests against the quality to the general chorus in the region. The vague and unconfirmed explanation going around seemed to be that this was the time of the year when the farmers were reaching the bottom of their silos, where the grain had been sitting for many months, and that when the new harvests came in from the fields, the situation would be relieved. Meanwhile, the grayish flour seemed to rise well, and there were no complaints about the taste. The brief flurry of illnesses at Connaux could have been the result of anything. With the hope that samples would immediately be lifted by the Union Meunière, the bakers had no choice but to continue blending the gray flour with their better stocks.

On Thursday, August 9, 1951, M. Bousquet squeezed his truck into Grande Rue at ten o'clock in the morning to supply M. Briand with seven sacks of flour from the mill of M. Maillet and eight from another mill. He continued his rounds at Pont-Saint-Esprit, delivering the same amounts to two other bakers of the village. M. Briand was ready with his protests as the delivery arrived, pointing out that the flour from M. Maillet's mill was certainly not of first quality and that something had to be done about it. He was perhaps more acutely aware than most bakers of the futility of his protest, because several years before he had refused to utilize a shipment of flour of obviously bad quality, and the prefecture had closed his shop down for a month.

On the following day, Friday, a fellow baker in the village, Marceau Benjamin Jaussent, called at M. Briand's shop to see if he could borrow two 100-kilo sacks of flour. Borrowing flour was a common practice among the bakers, especially since the Union Meunière demanded cash-on-delivery, and no longer extended a thirty-day billing period so the bakers could keep stock on hand and pay for it at the end of the month. It was about ten o'clock in the evening, and M. Briand was busy, as was his custom at this time, with the ovens. He gave M. Jaussent the key to the storeroom and told him to help himself.

M. Jaussent did not begin to "work" the borrowed flour until Saturday evening, the eleventh of August. As he began to work it, he thought that it smelled faintly of fuel oil. But other than that the flour was acceptable enough and compared favorably with the other stock he had on hand. He prepared only *une petite fournée*, or baking, that night, enough to supply Mme. Colonna with bread for sandwiches at her refreshment stand at Pont d'Ardèche, and a few other loaves for his own use.

At his own table that night, and later on Sunday, M. Jaussent and his family ate the bread and enjoyed it. It was not until late Sunday evening that his eleven-year-old son complained of feeling extremely cold in his hands and feet and later vomited considerably. On Monday morning his thirteen-year-old son and daughter began to have the same symptoms, as well as his wife. All broke out with a slight rash on their skins. By Wednesday M. Jaussent had joined them and was forced to go to bed for several days. Later, he learned that some of his clients complained of the same troubles. But the complaints, generally, were mild, and no one associated them directly with the bread. The news of the other *malades* from Connaux had not reached Pont-Saint-Esprit at that time, and the mild attacks were accepted with Gallic resignation.

On the evening of Wednesday, August 15, M. Briand stopped by the shop of M. Jaussent to see if the borrowed flour could be returned. He was greeted by M. Jaussent's father-in-law, who told Briand that Jaussent was not feeling too well, and was confined to his bed. However, it was perfectly all right for M. Briand to reclaim at least one sack of flour due him, and if he would send his helper, it would be immediately available. By half past eight in the evening, Aimé Pradier, M. Briand's helper, or *mitron*, had returned with the sack.

M. Briand and Pradier began to prepare three different batches of bread that night and morning. The first was out of the oven by three in the morning, and consisted of the flour Briand already had on hand. The second baking was not completed until about eight o'clock on Thursday morning, and was made from a mixture of the original flour and that taken back from M. Jaussent. Because of minor holidays at this time in August, the distribution center was closed, and M. Briand found that he had to borrow a second and third sack from two other local bakers that night. It was not until noon on Thursday, August 16, that the third and last baking was completed.

Most of the flour he was forced to use that night came from the mill of M. Maillet. M. Briand was not pleased with it. As he worked the dough, he noticed that it was slightly gray, but certainly no more so than the general supply that all the bakers were receiving. He tasted it several times to find it acceptable, if not equally as good as the normal flour received during the better seasons. He nevertheless resolved to lodge another protest, stronger this time, when the distribution center opened Friday morning, and then he went on with his work.

By nine o'clock Thursday morning, August 16, M. Briand was able to rest long enough to take a light meal on the counter of his shop. The bread was fresh, but no longer warm. The crust was crisp, and of the usual golden brown color. Its taste, to M. Briand's expert tongue, was good. Behind him the long, thin *baguettes*, the *gros pains*, larger and thicker, the *flûtes*, middle-sized, were stacked like soldiers at attention on the shelves. Night had run out, and already the first clients were beginning to arrive. One by one the shutters along Grande Rue were beginning to open. The sun of the Midi, already warm, was promising to broil later in the day. To the villagers, to the farmers nearby, to the workers in the vineyards, it was just another hot Languedoc-Provençal day. No one was prepared for what was going to happen. No one could be expected to be.

TWO

BY TEN O'CLOCK that Thursday morning all the shops along Grande Rue were welcoming their customers, the stone houses along the pavementless street giving some welcome shade from the August sun. Under the plane trees, some distance away, the *boules* players were gathered, most of them the older men of the village, already pensioned, with their retirement assured by the state. Their passion for *boules* was equaled only by their fondness for a milky glass of water and *pastis*, the aniseed alcohol drink so popular in Provence. The sandy gravel strip that divides the Boulevard Carnot from the rue de la Liberté served as the playing ground for the players, clustered in several groups along the strip. One by one they would toss out the small wooden target ball, *le bouchon* as it is called. And one by one, the players would throw the heavy metal balls, about the size and weight of ancient canon balls, and try to land nearer to the target than the others. Through it all, the groans and cheers of the spectators continued. Occasionally a player would wander away to the *tabac* for a package of Gauloise cigarettes, puffing a wreath of the sour smoke as he returned.

The workers in the village factory, which made the bottles for the sparkling Perrier water, by custom would be glancing at the clock to count off the moments until the long midday siesta. As in most of France, they would return to their homes for a sizable dinner in spite of the heat. But this day was different. They were out on strike, and dispersed among the *boules* players or off fishing to mark time until the strike was settled. At the village washing place, along the edge of the Rhône, the women were beating their laundry on the broad stone rim, chattering among themselves as their predecessors had done for centuries. The fresh, bright spring water ran freely through the large rectangular tanks of the municipal wash basins, just as it gushed from the gargoyles of the Fontaine de la Navigation and the swans of the Fontaine du Coq. Even the few women who had washing machines at times preferred to gather at the basin to rinse their wash, for there was much to talk about, especially the coming *Fête du Premier de Septembre,* only fifteen days away.

At the Café de la Bourse and the Café des Voyageurs, the sidewalk tables had already attracted their *habitués,* some of them sipping the bitter *café-filtre,* leavened by a sugar cube; some already getting a head start with a glass of *pastis.* The stone streets everywhere were hot, and no breeze was stirring to lighten the burden of the *Spiritpontains,* as the villagers call themselves.

Some housewives were shopping, and shopping is a serious business. They are immersed in their families, and to keep them clean and well fed is the limited dream of their lives. On this morning, as on any other morning, the *Spiritpontain* wives could be seen walking through the crooked streets with empty wine casks to fulfill their obligations as they gained the pleasure of the local news and gossip. They would be searching for arichide oil, rather than the insalubrious butter of the North, and *huile d'olive* for the sauces for salads and the traditional garlic soup. Here they would be boiling the garlic cloves in water, adding Gruyère cheese and cubes of toasted bread to soothe the overheated nerves of their husbands as they returned from the shops or vineyards at noontime.

In the houses the cool stone walls would be keeping the heat to a bearable level, while the wives would use their artistry with herbs and *vin courant* to convert a cheap cut of meat into a lordly meal. White wine to glorify the rabbit, red with other meats, along with thyme and bay leaves and whole cloves. On this morning, as on others, the *alimentation* shops remained Aladdin's caves for the fruit and vegetable shoppers, always demanding fresh greens for the midday repast, or any other meal. At the *charcuterie,* the sausages, hams, *saucissons, pâtés,* black pudding, and *caillettes*—small balls of mincemeat mixed with local grasses—were forcing the wives into agonizing decisions, tempered by the fact that regardless of the choice of meat, there was always the goats' cheese, wrapped in green leaves, to counterbalance any temporary dislike of the main *viande.*

And of course, the *boulangerie.* By ten that morning, the loaves of the first *fournée*—or baking—were almost gone from the shelves of M. Briand. Aimé Pradier, the eighteen-year-old helper of Briand had completed most of his chores, and had sat down for a moment to enjoy his *petit déjeuner,* including several generous slices from the second baking. By midday he joined his patron and family in their apartments adjoining the shop to eat his lunch, and the bread still hot from the ovens of the third scheduled baking of the day.

The headlines of the day were to be strangely familiar fifteen years later, though few in Pont-Saint-Esprit would be reading them: China was claiming total equality with the Soviet Union, and Mao was taking severe umbrage at the Soviets. The struggle in Vietnam was bitter and endless—but it was the French, of course, and not the United States, at that time. Only a few days before, a French general had been killed by a terrorist grenade in South Vietnam. The usual soccer and rugby matches between the villages were being played, and of course the bloody automobile accidents of the day were announced in screaming headlines.

On this morning, Mme. Eynard had more than usual to do, and rose early to get a head start on the day. There were the children to take care of, the household to supervise, and breakfast to prepare for her husband before he went to his *cabinet* to prepare for the long list of dental appointments for the day. In fact, the appointment schedule was so overcrowded that for the first time in several months, Mme. Eynard was planning to come in and assist with the dentistry to relieve some of the load from her husband. By the time Francine arrived to help with the household, Mme. Eynard was already behind schedule. She had planned to do her shopping before going to help her husband, including a visit to M. Briand's bakery on Grande Rue, which was in the same *quartier* of the village.

"I'm afraid I'm terribly late this morning," she told Francine. "If you would, I'd like you to do the shopping for the food and bread for me."

She went over the list with Francine, gave her the purse and shopping basket, and rushed off to join her husband at their offices. Francine, who patronized a different baker from M. Briand, went by habit to get the bread at her usual shop, not dreaming for a moment the significance of her act. On the way, however, she met her sister, Mme. Charpail, returning from the shop of M. Briand, and Francine regretted she had not bought the bread there because her sister told her that M. Briand was giving free bread to those workers who at the moment were out on strike at the factory. A baker who supported the workers should get her support, Francine thought. After all, her sister was one of the workers. Mme. Charpail said good-bye to Francine and returned to her home on the rue des Quatre Coins to enjoy a midmorning snack of bread and coffee. She had a passion for fresh bread, and her time off from the factory gave her an opportunity to eat some this morning, more oven-fresh than usual. Beside her, in the cradle, her nine-month-old baby girl gurgled peacefully.

Over three hundred people in the village bought their bread that day at M. Briand's shop. M. Carle, whose grocery shop was considered by many to be the finest in town, sent his maid to bring back three loaves for lunch and dinner that day, although usually he patronized another baker, whose shop was closed for the holidays. M. Sauvet, a garageman in the village also patronized another baker, but today M. Carle's small daughter volunteered to go to the store for him and his wife, and finding their customary bakery closed, brought back two loaves of bread from M. Briand.

There were others who bought their bread from M. Briand who never had before; there were some who, by fate or accident, bought their bread this day from another *boulangerie*, although they had patronized M. Briand on every other day.

Mme. Paul Rieu dropped by the shop of M. Briand in the late

morning. She and her husband were fond of the bread Briand had been baking so many years in the town, and she exchanged pleasantries with Mme. Briand, who helped behind the counter during the busy times of the day, as well as their daughter Yvonne. All through the day the front door opened and closed endlessly. The clients came not from Pont-Saint-Esprit alone, but from many of the surrounding villages: from Saint-Julien-de-Peyrolas, from the Route d'Ardèche, from Carsan, from Saint-Paulet-de-Caisson, from Saint Alexandre. There was Joseph Puche, the ex-pilot, and Louis Guigou, the *garagiste,* and Mme. Boudenne, wife of the genial proprietor of the local hat-and-sporting-goods store, Marcel Boudenne. On the Grande Rue the neighbors filed in and out, with brief but newsy exchanges of greetings: Mme. Brahic, Mme. Chambon, Marie Baverel, Jean Crebier, Blanche Morgan, Mme. Payan, and Hélène Charrière, wife of the pharmacist on the street. Carefully, they would choose the loaves of their liking, whether *flûte, baguette,* or *gros pain,* marching out on the hot street with the unwrapped bread under their arms or strapped across the back of a bicycle.

At noon on that day M. Marcel Delacquis was at work at his desk at the Coopérative des Céréales de Pont-Saint-Esprit. As manager of the organization his days were filled with the endless details of receiving and shipping grain and fertilizers for the farmers in the region, and he almost forgot that he had promised to bring the bread back to Mme. Testevin at the villa where he was a *pensionnaire,* or boarder.

Shortly after twelve he stopped his dictation to Mlle. Wullschleger, his secretary, and dismissed her with apologies for running over into the lunch hour. M. Delacquis was a precise and intelligent man, an artist and poet of measurable talent as well as a man of commerce. Some of his poems had appeared in a national anthology of French poets. He did not like to impose on those who worked for him, and his sensitivity and consideration was marked and admired by all who had dealings with him. As a Parisian with considerable travel and work abroad, he was somewhat of an anomaly in Pont-Saint-Esprit. But his quiet, self-effacing demeanor enabled him to blend into the customs of the village soundlessly. After serving in World War I, he had become a sales representative in Argentina, and worked in that area for several different French companies, whose products included school supplies, lace, religious art, and gloves. It was his health that had prompted him to give up a life of travel and the pressures of Paris to retire to less demanding work in the Provençal atmosphere.

His accommodations at La Villette, the large farmhouse of the Testevin family, enabled him to enjoy the country air yet still remain within a kilometer of his office in the village. He had a large bedroom in one corner of the villa, looking out on the courtyard and the vineyards beyond. The room was furnished modestly in French provincial style, and the rich red tile floor was cooling in the heat of the summer days. On the walls he had hung a few of his paintings—soft, sensitive oils of the surrounding countryside in subdued and restrained colors. As in all the other rooms in La Villette, a crucifix hung on the wall.

After straightening up his desk, he locked the office door for the long two-hour midday siesta and pedaled off on his bicycle down the rue de l'Ouest and along the Boulevard Gambetta. Turning into Grande Rue and proceeding to the shop of M. Briand, he parked his bicycle outside and entered to greet Mme. Briand, who was behind the counter. After an exchange of pleasantries he asked for two *gros pains*—loaves weighing about a kilo each, a little over two pounds. Mme. Briand did not have any left on the shelves and went to the back of the store to get them. She returned promptly with the two loaves and passed them across the counter to him. He paid the money, fifty old francs, and went out to put them into the sack tied to his bicycle. One reason he preferred to buy his bread from M. Briand was that the baker supplied him with a special sack for his bicycle. He pedaled slowly back along Grande Rue, which by now was nearly deserted, for the shops were closed and the villagers had retreated to their houses for the almost sacred midday repast.

La Villette, a stone and plaster *mas*, as a large farmhouse is called in the Midi, rests on a high hill overlooking Pont-Saint-Esprit. A long stone work shed extends out from one side of the house, and an ornate iron gate marks the entrance. One side without windows faces the direction of the mistral, which blows and screeches during the fall, winter, and spring months and at times frays the nerves of everyone. Mme. Testevin took in selected boarders, mothered them, and fed them with lavish attention. At that time in 1951 the house was not as famous as later, when it came to be known as the birthplace of Jacqueline Kennedy's great-grandfather. Later, all of Pont-Saint-Esprit would bathe in the reflected fame of the Bouvier family, after Jacqueline Kennedy became the First Lady of the White House. Mme. Testevin, proud to be a cousin of the Bouvier family, not only managed the full household, but helped her husband with the vineyards, took care of the laundry, and grew many of her own herbs and vegetables. M. Testevin, a ruddy, lean, and tall farmer in his fifties, tended twenty-five thousand vines with care and passion and produced eighty thousand litres of wine each year.

M. Delacquis, puffing up the hill on his bicycle, reached Mme. Testevin's kitchen barely in time for the luncheon ritual.

At the table was the usual group found these days at La Villette. M. Testevin was at the head of the long farmhouse table, Mme. Testevin at the other end, near the kitchen. On one side, with their backs to the window, sat Emile Cima—a genial Italian worker in the vineyards, a man strong as an ox but soft in manner—and M. Delacquis, the slim and soft-mannered Parisian. Opposite them sat Mme. Dezeuzes, a gentle lady living at the farm in the room next to the Testevin quarters. The men, freshly in from the vineyards, ate heartily of the *pot-au-feu,* the thick vegetable soup with large chunks of beef in which Mme. Testevin prided herself. The others ate less avariciously, but savored the flavor, for it was good. The large carafes of red and rose wine came from their own vineyards, and each helped himself freely, under M. Testevin's urging. Nearly all enjoyed the Provençal custom of dipping large chunks of bread in the stew, and the meal was finished off with goats' cheese, Gruyére, and a heaping bowl of fruit. The conversation was light and pleasant, for this was a *gentil* group, courteous, and sensitive to the needs of the others.

Scores of other tables in or near the village of Pont-Saint-Esprit were served with much the same type of meal, with minor variations. In other homes there were eggs *soufflé,* or *salade Niçoise,* or *omelettes aux fines herbes,* or *potage de légumes,* or *bifteck,* or thrush liver, known as *pâté de grives.* Whatever the course, the bread played a large part of the meal.

No one at any table in the region that day made any complaint about the taste of M. Briand's bread. M. Delacquis, more used to the whiteness of Parisian bread, felt that it was perhaps a little gray in color, but the flavor was good. Emile, robust and tanned from the vineyards, ate more heartily than the others, for his appetite matched his strength. M. Testevin, too, ate heavily to fortify himself against the long, hot afternoon. Mme. Testevin ate only a slice no bigger than her little finger.

By quarter of two in the afternoon the group had dispersed, content with the repast. Mme. Testevin cleared the table, Mme. Dezeuzes retired to her room. Emile and M. Testevin excused themselves and moved out into the vineyards, which were within weeks of being harvested. M. Delacquis mounted his bicycle again and coasted off toward his office in the village. For all at this table, and for the others in the area, another ordinary summer midday meal had come to an end.

Shortly after the noon hour had begun, M. Briand prepared, as was his custom, to make his delivery rounds in the surrounding countryside. He gathered his loaves together, for there were several large *domaines* in the outlying section with working crews and large families who counted on his deliveries. Among them were the Moulin and Mison families, living out in the country near Carsan. The *domaine* of Joseph Moulin was particularly far out, and the baker left his loaves for the Moulins at a neighboring farm. After several other deliveries he returned to his shop to prepare, as usual, for the bakings the next day, Friday, August 17. He had not been back in the shop more than an hour or so before Felix Mison, the farmer from Carsan, entered to chide him mildly for forgetting to drop off his customary order of bread. M. Briand suddenly realized he had forgotten the delivery and quickly apologized. M. Mison accepted the apologies in good humor, paid for the bread, and left the shop. Once again M. Briand and the village itself settled down to its usual midweek routine.

On his vacation in the Pyrenees, some five hundred miles away, Dr. Albert Gabbai, one of the three physicians in Pont-Saint-Esprit, was facing an entirely different type of weather on that day: rain. In fact, it had rained almost constantly since he and his family had been away—over a week. It was not the kind of weather fit for a holiday, and after a great deal of thought during the day his family finally agreed with him that it would be better if he went home ahead of the rest of the family and made up the remaining days of his vacation in more seasonable weather. Mme. Gabbai helped him pack, and he phoned ahead to his *femme de ménage* to indicate that he would be coming back on the following day, Friday.

The drive back was long and tiring. He left the mountains at five in the morning, pacing himself so that he would not have to hurry in the face of the tourist traffic that plied all summer long on the route through Pont-Saint-Esprit, a main route toward the Spanish border. The road, brushing near the rich historical centers of Arles, Pont-du-Gard, Les Baux, Beaucaire, Tarascon-sur-Rhône, Nîmes, Montpellier, Carcasonne, and others, made it a favorite for tourists, and created heavy traffic problems. He planned to reach home before dinner. He hoped that it would be waiting for him as he had arranged. As Dr. Gabbai was driving his car on the long route home, back in Pont-Saint-Esprit, M. Briand was at last receiving another shipment of flour from M. Bousquet so that he would be able to return the borrowed sacks he had been using during the time when he was unable to get delivery. For two days now he had worked almost exclusively with the gray flour from the north, and he did not relish the idea of continuing that way, at least without some whiter flour to blend with it. He was disappointed when M. Bousquet informed him that he would have to take along, with a dozen other sacks, at least six or seven of the bags of northern flour—there was nothing else that could be delivered. M. Bousquet was nervous and edgy, because this was the day the mayor of Saint-Génies-de-Comolas had visited him, and he was now holding off pressures on all sides. He tossed Briand's empty sacks into his truck with the sacks of other bakers, to return to the Union Meuniére. He tried to avoid direct answers to Briand's penetrating questions about the quality. M. Bousquet had already written his bitter letter of complaint to his superiors at Nîmes that morning, and was doing everything that could be done under the distribution system of the Union Meunière.

The *domaine* of Joseph Moulin stretched across the rolling foothills of the Massif Central for hundreds of acres. The vines in the rich Rhône soil were cared for with affection and love, for M. Moulin was a perfectionist, and his *domaine* was considered among the finest in the region. It had been in the family since 1789, a testimony to the continuous diligence of the family through the generations. Although they were only a few kilometers from Pont-Saint-Esprit, his vineyards seemed remote from all of civilization, for not another house was visible, except in the far distance. The vines were rich and full that August of 1951, and both M. Moulin and his wife Laurain were happy and proud to see that young Joseph, at the age of twenty-five, was taking over more and more of the responsibility for managing the meticulous and infinite chores necessary to bring the grapes to maturity. There is almost a spiritual quality to the raising of fine grapes in France, and young Joseph was beginning to show this quality more each day. What is more, he was liked by all the young men and women of Pont-Saint-Esprit, a favorite among them for his zest for living, his high good humor, his strength and affection. Young Joseph was *sérieux*, as the French say about those who are solid and substantial citizens.

He was respected by the men who worked for him in the vineyards. In Provence and Languedoc the sun and the mistral are enemies, and the art of growing grapes requires both strength and cunning to avoid their savage attacks. Young Joseph already had learned how to use both, and he inspired the workers to do likewise. The people in the village liked to talk about the time young Joseph found a worker unwilling to try to lift a sack of nitrate fertilizer onto a truck. He placed the sack in the arms of the worker, it was said, and lifted both to the back of the truck in one smooth motion.

At lunchtime on Friday, August 17, young Joseph had come in from the vineyards with a ravenous hunger. He ate unsparingly of Mme. Moulin's *bouillon gras*—a tasty, thin stew for warm weather—which pleased his mother greatly. His 213-pound frame needed nourishment, she felt, and she constantly went out of her way to cook the things he liked. He also ate the bread, nearly a full *gros pain*, before his hunger gave in. It was the bread M. Briand had delivered the day before on his rounds at Carsan. The seven workers at the table also ate heavily, for they enjoyed Mme. Moulin's table as much as young Joseph did.

There was still some bread left that night after dinner, and as was her custom, Mme. Moulin fed the scraps to the cat, the ducks, and the dog. Strangely enough the dog leaped to the platter on the kitchen floor, rushed through the remains of the *bouillon gras* without hesitation, but only sniffed at and backed away from the bread. Since he had never rejected bread before, Mme. Moulin tasted again the small chunk remaining in her hand, but found nothing wrong with it, except perhaps that it seemed flatter than usual, she thought.

The Moulin family retired early that Friday night, after the same dinnertime menu that had been followed at lunch. The heat of the Midi sun stayed on through the night, which was without a stirring of air. At the time when you need the mistral, many Provençals have said, it will never blow. In his room young Joseph Moulin awoke at some indistinguishable hour of the night with sharp, colicky pains in his stomach. They made him uncomfortable, but he had had worse pains, and he finally fell back asleep, in exhaustion from his work in the fields and vineyards.

In the morning he felt better. There were no complaints from the others, although Mme. Moulin told them how strange it was the dog had rejected the bread in the *bouillon gras*. Father and son chided her, ate their *petit déjeuner*, and went out to join the work crew already waiting for them.

Cleaning up the kitchen, Mme. Moulin was stopped short by an utterly strange and sharp cry from the cat. She looked down on the floor, as the cat screamed in agony again. Then it rolled over, writhed, twisted, shook, and ran screaming toward the wall, trying to climb it. Its hair was literally standing up on end. She ran to it, tried to pick it up, to comfort it, but it hissed and spit at her, then screamed in the most unearthly sound she had ever heard. Alone in the house, she had no one to turn to, and all her efforts to pick up the cat were hopeless. Again and again it batted itself against the wall, then rolled on the floor in convulsions. It was a hideous, frightening sight, she later said, shocking beyond belief. Unable to climb the wall now, it ran into it at blinding speed, as if it were intent on self-destruction. In tears, Mme. Moulin coaxed, and pleaded with the cat to come to her, but each time was repulsed. Then with another terrifying scream, clawing wildly at the air, it dropped to the tiles, motionless. In a moment it pulled itself up on its forelegs, then dragged its hind legs across the floor, collapsing again next to the stove.

At this moment Mme. Moulin looked out the open kitchen door to the barnyard. One duck was lying prostrate on its side. Another was staggering, as if drunk, beside it. Three others were clacking ceaselessly, their bills stretched as if they were going to break. They were marching and strutting like penguins, flapping their wings and waddling in a most unnatural way. From the doorway Mme. Moulin watched them in awe. She had been brought up on a *mas*, lived all her life among domestic animals. She had never seen anything like this, ever. The three lively ducks were now reaching a crescendo in their quacking and their strutting. Their waddling became more exaggerated, their likeness to penguins even more pronounced. She crossed over the gravel yard to the prostrate duck and lifted his head. It fell back limply. The second was by then turning slowly in circles, then it dropped also. The others continued their wild chorus. She looked anxiously out over the vineyards, but her husband and son and the workers were nowhere in sight. Terrified, she ran back into the kitchen. The cat had not moved from where it had fallen. Carefully, slowly, she picked it up. It was dead.

Not far away, in the same village of Carsan, Félix Mison was feeding the leftover bread to his dog, a chore he enjoyed along with his work as a *cultivateur* in the region. A quiet and well-liked farmer, he had built up over the years a prosperous and well-tended farm, raised a happy and contented family. After the dog had wolfed down the chunks, M. Mison played with him affectionately, throwing a stick out to be retrieved, roughing up his fur, and accepting a few friendly licks on the ear.

Three hours later the dog limply rose from the kitchen floor, whimpering strangely. It moved out to the farmyard, M. Mison following in astonishment. He had never seen it act this way before. About twenty feet away from the door, the dog stopped in its tracks, leaped grotesquely in the air, and began running swiftly in a wide circle. M. Mison tried futilely to stop him, but each time he got near the dog, it snarled and snapped at him viciously. At moments the dog would seize a rock, crunch it fiercely in its teeth until at last two teeth fell out, and blood dripped from its mouth. For nearly ten minutes the macabre scene continued; Mme. Mison now joined her husband to try to calm the animal. Running more slowly now, dragging its motionless back legs, it finally wobbled to a hollow in the dirt and sunk down in it. Its breathing was labored and heavy, and the dry blood was caked in its mouth. Within the hour, it, too, was dead.

The dog had been a favorite of the family. Its death affected the Misons severely. So much so that M. Mison almost failed to notice the gripping pains in his own stomach, which had begun shortly after the dog had died. Perhaps, thought M. Mison, this was a reaction to the loss of his pet. He lay down on his bed, in sorrow, pain, and puzzlement.

Friday evening at La Villette was a festive one for the Testevin family and their *pensionnaires*. Friends from Toulon, laden with gifts and food, arrived in happy spirits, glad to visit the country, away from the noise and clatter of the city. They brought their own bread, a common custom in France, and presented Mme. Testevin with a mess of *truite de rivière*, brown trout freshly caught from the Rhône, and a bottle of *pastis*. M. and Mme. Lamacchir were jewelers, longtime friends of the Testevins, and they brightened the dinner table that evening with tales of life in their coastal city of Toulon, as M. Delacquis spoke of his travels in South America. The trout, smothered in almonds and olive oil, was cooked to a crisp brown turn by Mme. Testevin. They lingered over the dinner a long time, sipping the wine and *pastis*. The Lamacchir's ate their own bread from Toulon, while the rest of the table finished up the bread of M. Briand, supplemented that afternoon with more loaves from his shop on the Grande Rue. After a short session of cards M. Delacquis excused himself and climbed the narrow stone stairs of the old house to his quarters. He read the paper for a brief time, then prepared for bed. He fell asleep quickly, but shortly after two in the morning he awoke feeling extremely nauseous. He now regretted having eaten the trout at dinner, delicious as it had been. In addition he found himself inexplicably chilly, although the night was warm and had cooled off little from the August day. He got up, went to his closet to fetch another blanket, but found himself shivering under it. He was unable to sleep, and also unable to vomit, in spite of the strong feeling of nausea.

It was not long after he had crawled, shivering, under the

blanket that he heard others in the house stirring. It was clear from the sounds in the Testevin room that Mme. Testevin was sick, and he tried to get up again to see if he could help. Weakness prevented him from rising, but he was convinced now that the trout had caused trouble not only with him, but with the rest of the household. He lay there awake and shivering through the night until the sun came up.

About two hours before the Testevin household sat down to their festive dinner on Friday evening, Dr. Albert Gabbai arrived at his home. He pulled his car into his courtyard, stretched as he got out of the car, and went into his house. It had been a long, tiring trip. He was greeted by the *femme de ménage,* who told him that his waiting room was filled with people, some of them referred by Dr. Vieu, who had learned that Dr. Gabbai was returning from vacation, and whose office was unusually overcrowded that day.

In the waiting room were nearly a dozen patients. Dr. Gabbai was astonished, but regained his composure and called in the first patient. He was the head of a family of thirteen people, with seven members sick from severe stomach trouble. When Dr. Gabbai learned that the six other members of the family were in the waiting room, he had them file into his office one by one for a necessarily quick examination. Their complaints were identical: stomach upset, nausea, chills. They had no fever; in fact most of the children and the father were experiencing *hypothermie,* their temperatures being measurably below normal.

None of them was seriously ill, but the fact that so many in one family were sick indicated the possibility of a mild poisoning, and would have to be investigated thoroughly. What had they eaten the night before? Most important: Had they all eaten the same thing? When the doctor was assured that the entire family had shared the exact same food, his puzzlement mounted. How could seven members suffer from food poisoning, while the other six experienced no trouble whatever?

He questioned the father in minute detail for nearly fifteen minutes. Nothing was revealed that could explain why nearly half the family remained perfectly healthy in the face of apparent food poisoning in the other half. The meat was served from a casserole.

Were there two casseroles at the table? No. Was any fish course served? No. Were any chemicals kept in the household? No. The questioning seemed to be futile. How about the seating arrangement? Was there any relation to this and the way the food was served?

The father hesitated a moment here. He recalled now that half the family sat on one side of the table and the other half on the other. Yes, there was a definite seating arrangement. Thinking carefully now, he reconstructed this in his mind. Not only was there a definite seating arrangement, but, yes, all the children with him in Dr. Gabbai's office were seated on one side of the table. There was no question about it.

But what had they eaten that those on the other side of the table had not? Ostensibly, nothing. Going back to the original question, those at the table had shared exactly the same food, and there seemed to be no logical explanation for the clear division between the sick and the well in the family.

The lack of logic for the situation plagued Dr. Gabbai. He prescribed a mild ameliorative for the stomach upsets and arranged to stop by the family's house the first available moment. In the meantime he requested the father to keep whatever leftovers remained from the food of the night before. The family filed out of the office, and Dr. Gabbai called in the next patient.

He was M. Guigou, a garage-owner in the village, another patient referred by Dr. Vieu because of the latter's overcrowded office. M. Guigou presented the same symptoms as the first patients. He was older, weaker, and less resilient. He had, he explained, eaten his meal, as was his habit, at the *pension* where he lived in the village, the Hôtel Redortier. Were any others at the hotel stricken with stomach upset? M. Guigou did not think so. What was served? Nothing particularly suspect. Did he eat anything that the others did not? The answer was negative.

Again, Dr. Gabbai was faced with an enigma. He prescribed a similar mild remedy, but ordered M. Guigou to bed immediately because of his age, then made a note to stop by the Hôtel Redortier to see what might be unearthed regarding the food served there the night before.

The dinner to which Dr. Gabbai had been looking forward all through the long drive back from the Pyrenees was ready, but it grew cold as more patients filed into the office, all with similar complaints. Some felt giddy, as if they had drunk too much wine, but they had drunk no more than usual. Some vomited. Some had diarrhea. Many had chills, reflected by subnormal temperatures. But none seemed seriously ill. When he collapsed into bed at eleven that night, Dr. Gabbai was confident that the worst was over, and that the town would return to normal in the morning.

When morning came, Dr. Gabbai's fears lessened. Reports from the patients of the day before indicated that they felt much better, for the most part. A telephone consultation with Dr. Vieu indicated the same conditions: The patients he had seen on Friday were showing marked signs of improvement, although his phone was already being clogged with new patients, suffering from the same symptoms. There was comfort in realizing that the attacks were apparently mild and benign, but it was important to try to track down the cause as soon as possible to prevent such an annoyance and nuisance from breaking out again. Dr. Vieu confessed to feeling shaky and ill himself, yet he felt he could not pinpoint the cause to anything particular that he had eaten the day before. Further, Dr. Channac, the third doctor in town, was definitely ill, which created a temporary extra load on Dr. Vieu and Dr. Gabbai. However, there was every indication that the new flurry of patients would subside, just as the first had. Meanwhile the two doctors agreed there was nothing much to do but grin and bear it. They agreed to check back with each other later in the day, as soon as they had the chance to try to investigate the cause of the nuisance.

Dr. Gabbai's first house call that Saturday morning was the result of an urgent request from Francine, sister of Mme. Charpail, who reported that the latter was seriously ill with symptoms that she had never before witnessed. During the night Mme. Charpail had a major fit of convulsions: Her eyes reversed in her head, her mouth foamed, saliva drained from her mouth, her features became unrecognizable. She was mute and silent now, and she had been moved downstairs to the rooms of her mother on the rue de Quatre Coins, so care could be taken of her nine-month-old baby.

Dr. Gabbai lost no time in reaching the house, where he found Mme. Charpail in another fit of convulsions. They subsided quickly after he arrived. The symptoms here were clear and unmistakable. They showed every sign of being those of *une crise d'épilepsie*. Yet what was most puzzling was the fact that there was no history whatever of epilepsy in the patient, and it would be extremely rare for a patient to have reached her twentieth birthday, which was the age of Mme. Charpail, without having manifested any symptoms before. For the second time in as many days he was faced with a major mystery. Another possibility was tetanus, but he could find no infection anywhere. Although he could see absolutely no relationship between the case of Mme. Charpail and his patients of the day before, he inquired at length about what food had been eaten in the household. There was nothing particularly suspect, although Mme. Charpail's mother pointed out that she had eaten a piece of melon the day before, which had been the only food Mme. Charpail had eaten that the rest of the family had not. The remains of the melon, however, had already been thrown out, and there were no means of checking into this as a possibility for the cause of the attack. Further, the symptoms did not seem to relate to food poisoning. The doctor indicated that he would keep Mme. Charpail under observation, and return later in the day.

At the household of the large family who had first visited his office, the doctor was relieved to find that those who had been sick were in better health. He again studied the situation of the suspected meal two evenings before. He verified that the seven members of the family who had become ill had sat on one side of the table; and the six who were untouched by any sickness had sat opposite them. But still no one could recall any special way the food was served so that nearly half would be stricken and the other half remain unscathed. Then one of the children remembered an important thing: She had been sent to the bakery to get one loaf of bread, which had not been enough; when she went out to get a second loaf, she went to a different bakery, the shop of M. Briand. Now she recalled clearly that those who fell ill had all sat on the side of the table where M. Briand's bread had been served. Slowly, several other members of the family were able to recall that this must have been true. They were not certain, however. The puzzle still remained, but a definite clue had been obtained. Dr. Gabbai took samples of some of the portions of the food that remained and brought them back to his office. Analysis of the food would have to wait until it could reach a laboratory.

He was greeted on his return with the same overcrowded waiting room. His *femme de ménage* told him that his phone had been ringing constantly with many calls from both the village and the surrounding country areas. Among them was a call from Mme. Mison in Carsan, who said that her husband was in severe pain and asked if the doctor could possibly come as soon as possible.

After treating those in his waiting room, all of whom were mildly ill with the same persistent complaints, Dr. Gabbai got into his car and drove as quickly as possible to the farmhouse of M. Mison. He was greeted at the door by Mme. Mison, who was embarrassed to say that her husband was now much better and that it must have been just a simple attack of indigestion. She apologized profusely for asking him to come all this distance for a false alarm. Dr. Gabbai, known to all the people in the region as a warm and generous person, reassured her and went to the bedside of her husband.

He was sitting up in bed now and no longer in pain. His symptoms were the usual ones, which Dr. Gabbai had by now come to expect of every patient he was treating. M. Mison protested that his wife should not have called him, that he had tried to persuade her not to do so. After the examination Dr. Gabbai was able to assure him that on the basis of the other patients with the same symptoms, he should be feeling much better soon. But the doctor wanted to know just what he had eaten in the last two days—especially, where had he bought the bread? M. Mison then related the story of how M. Briand usually delivered the bread to his farm and of how the delivery had not arrived on Thursday afternoon. He went on to explain his call at M. Briand's shop, how he had softly chided M. Briand for forgetting the delivery, and how he had bought and carried the bread back to his house himself. Now a second piece of evidence suggesting that it might have been the bread had come to the attention of Dr. Gabbai. After prescribing some medicine for M. Mison, he left at once to finish up his investigation. He felt at last he was getting somewhere, even though full proof was yet to come. Just after he left, the Misons remembered a disquieting thing: They had forgotten to tell him of the sad and tragic death of their dog, who—they recalled now with sharp and sudden horror—had died shortly after eating the same bread.

When he got back to town, Dr. Gabbi tried to reach Dr. Vieu, but without success. He then stopped by the town hall to notify the authorities that a mild outbreak of food poisoning seemed to be evident. He was asked to report more facts, and an investigation was immediately promised by the mayor of the village.

From the town hall he went to the Hôtel Redortier to visit M. Guigou, who was feeling in better spirits and seemed to be shaking off the annoying symptoms of the previous day. But here another clear piece of evidence was contributed: Pressed about where the bread he ate came from, M. Guigou related that he always brought his own bread to the hotel, bread he always bought at the shop of M. Briand. He was the only one of the ten boarders who ate the bread and the only one who was ill.

The doctor returned to his office, notified the mayor's office that the bread of M. Briand was definitely suspect, and once again tried in vain to reach Dr. Vieu, who was himself so busy making his rounds that he could not get back to his office.

It was not until eleven o'clock on Saturday evening that Dr. Vieu and Dr. Gabbai were able to meet in the latter's office to compare notes.

The facts added up to rather alarming proportions, somewhat mollified, however, by the mildness of the illness, which by now both doctors were certain could be attributed to the bread of M. Briand.

Between them the two doctors counted some 230 patients in Pont-Saint-Esprit, and in the surrounding villages and countryside.

Nausea, vomiting, and diarrhea were among the most constant symptoms.

Hypothermie, subnormal temperature, was almost universal. This was accompanied by severe shivering, in spite of the hot August temperatures.

Many cases of slow pulse, *bradycardie,* were noted.

Enlargement of the pupils, *mydriase,* was also evident in many cases.

A large proportion exhibited *angoisse*, severe difficulty in breathing.

Because of the impossibly overloaded schedule of both doctors, neither was able to make a complete and intelligent analysis of the over-all picture. Independently, they had arrived at the conclusion that M. Briand's bread was the source of the trouble. Neither had had a single patient who had *not* eaten the bread out of the shop on Grande Rue. In fact, nearly all residents on Grande Rue, habitual buyers of M. Briand's bread, were sick with the key symptoms to a greater or lesser degree. The only encouraging thing about the situation was the fact that the symptoms were still mild, and seemed to be clearing up after the initial attacks were over.

Even though it was late at night, both doctors went to see Mayor Hebrard at his home. The first action seemed clear and obvious: Every bakery in town should be closed pending a further and immediate investigation by the police. The doctors would continue to accept any patient they encountered regardless of whose patient he normally was. The news that Dr. Channac was recovering from his illness was an encouraging and hopeful sign, because both Dr. Vieu and Dr. Gabbai were beginning to show signs of exhaustion.

All three looked forward to Sunday morning, since there was reason to believe the worst was over. Both Dr. Vieu and Dr. Channac, who had eaten the bread themselves, were already beginning to feel better after their initial discomfort.

On Saturday morning, before the doctors had begun their strange and exhausting day, M. Delacquis rose at his usual hour at La Villette, feeling slightly better than he had during the night. He was not, oddly enough, at all tired, even though he had no sleep at all after his attack had struck him. Downstairs in the big country kitchen Mme. Testevin was already at work. Both agreed that the trout must have been the cause of their uncomfortable night, for it seemed that everyone in the household, except the visitors from Toulon, had been sick. Neither M. Testevin nor Emile had slept, yet both had already gone out to work in the vineyards. M. Delacquis and Mme. Testevin agreed that everyone would probably feel better after the effects had worn off, later on in the day.

The guests, who seemed to have escaped illness, were still asleep.

M. Delacquis cycled down the hill to the village in another burning Midi day and arrived at the Coopérative des Céréales de Pont-Saint-Esprit promptly at eight o'clock. Aside from his feeling lightheaded, the disturbances of the previous night did not seem to linger with him. Saturday at the office was always a busy day, because it was necessary to make out all the checks for the farmers' wheat and grain payments and wind up the affairs of the week. Mlle. Wullschleger was already there when he arrived, and they sat down to tackle the endless details of the routine. All the records of the shipments and receipts for each client had to be adjusted according to the weights registered on the scales during the previous week, and the checks that were prepared for each client required innumerable small calculations. It was painstaking work. During the process M. Delacquis began to find a strange dizziness coming over him, which he tried desperately to shake. He said nothing about it to Mlle. Wullschleger, but she began to note the fact that M. Delacquis was not feeling at all well, and she asked him about it.

"I'm sure," he told her, "that it must be the trout we ate last night. Nearly everyone in the house felt the same way last night."

"Perhaps," said Mlle. Wullschleger, "I could take some of the work off your hands."

"It will take all day for the two of us to finish the job," he said. "I couldn't let you do that."

The checks were the most important item on the agenda that morning, and they concentrated on those. But by a quarter of twelve, the checks were less than half prepared. The president of the cooperative arrived at that moment, and expecting the task to be completed was astonished to find that the job was taking so long. There was a heated discussion. M. Delacquis, rising to cross to the file, found that he could not get up from the chair and fell back in it. The room began to spin, and he found it necessary to squeeze the arms of the chair to keep his equilibrium. He told the president, who was nervous and impatient, that he would return early from lunch and that the checks would be completed by midafternoon, only a few hours behind schedule. Reassured, the president left the office.

M. Delacquis found the dizzy spell subsiding and decided that perhaps he would feel stronger after lunch. He was able to get up now, and he crossed the office to the door without difficulty. Mlle. Wullschleger tried to assist him, but he refused her help.

"I'll be perfectly all right," he said, "as soon as I get something in my stomach."

Mlle. Wullschleger, worried, watched him from the door. She knew that he was a stubborn and determined man when he wanted to be, and that it was useless to offer him further help. She watched as he mounted his bicycle, and even though he had some difficulty mounting it, he began pedaling down the road, with the bicycle wobbling beneath him. "God help him make it," she said to herself. She knew instinctively that he would not be returning that afternoon.

The ride up the hill to La Villette seemed a million miles to M. Delacquis. The road seemed to shrink and expand in front of his eyes. The villas along the side of the road took on brilliant and indescribable colors. When he looked down at his hands on the handlebars, they seemed to stretch miles in front of him. The road would widen out to infinity, and then return to a size no larger than a ribbon. The front wheel of his bicycle would begin to grow until it seemed to encompass the entire world, and suddenly it would return to normal. He had a strange feeling of being outside himself, as if he were looking down at the figure pumping so laboriously up the hill. The journey seemed to be taking him centuries, yet at the same time he seemed to be moving at an incredible speed, whisking on the wings of a magic carpet past the vineyards, which were no longer ordinary vineyards, but blazing rows of glorious colors. He seemed to float in time and space, and as he entered the courtyard of La Villette, he felt he was borne in on the wings of a mythical golden chariot.

Mme. Testevin, at the washing well of the courtyard, saw him come. It was a pitiful, painful sight. His bicycle was wobbling dizzily over the rough gravel. His face was strained, pale, and pinched. She ran toward him, because she knew he was going to fall, but she was too late. Near the old well his bicycle spun crazily out from under him to the left, while he spun off to the right onto the dirt. Breathing heavily, he lay limply on the ground. She helped him to his feet, and he seemed to recover his equilibrium quickly. Painfully, with her help, he made his way to his room. By the time they reached it, he was already feeling much better. He refused to let her send someone for the doctor, because he was certain now that the worst was over. He begged her not to be concerned, explaining that this must be a new form of his older illness, which had made him leave Paris and come to the country. If by the next morning, Sunday, he did not feel better, he agreed he would let her call the doctor.

Fully clothed, he collapsed on the bed in exhaustion.

THREE

On Saturday, before the doctors had begun to suspect that bread was the source of the ailments that were coming to their attention, M. Briand worked in his shop as usual. He had no inkling that his bread had anything whatever to do with the fact that he had not been able to sleep for twenty-four hours, and that his wife, his helper, and he himself were feeling mildly upset with stomach trouble, as so many others in the village were feeling. Events grow slowly; those facts that emerge clearly and unmistakably in hindsight are often muddled and obscure in the early beginnings. It is only after the small links of the chain are assembled that any kind of a picture begins to emerge. Further, the beginnings of a tragedy are often infinitely small, undiscernible in the everyday pressures of ordinary life. On that Saturday people were almost totally unaware that many others were feeling liverish, and since the symptoms were so mild, little talk took place in the village streets that day.

To M. Briand, the mild upset experienced by him and his family could have been the result of any number of things, and because of its lightness, it was barely worth thinking about. Hardly anyone in the village was comparing notes, and those who did, shrugged off their complaints, as most people do with the minor annoyances of living.

M. Briand, for instance, was preoccupied with a trip to the Ardèche River, where two of his children were on vacation. He and his wife left almost at dawn early Sunday morning. They were pleased to be away from the routine of the week and were looking forward to greeting their children along the pleasant wooded banks of the river, where the heat of the bakery and the village streets could be forgotten. His wife was feeling slightly better, and the only unusual thing he noticed was that he had not been able to sleep again for a second night, yet he felt completely refreshed and vigorous, ready to enjoy their brief respite.

Just a few hours before M. Briand left for the Ardèche, in the early dark hours on Sunday morning, the phone of Dr. Gabbai rang again.

Mme. Mison's voice was trembling now; she was obviously fighting to keep down panic. "It's my husband again," she said. "He is terribly ill now. Terribly. He can hardly breathe, hardly talk. Please, Doctor. I know you must be exhausted. But is there anything that can be done? Anything? I forgot to tell you—our dog died after eating the bread. Does that . . . that have anything to do with this?"

Within minutes Dr. Gabbai was dressed and getting into his car. The streets of the village were black and silent. He streaked along the Boulevard Gambetta, past the Hôtel de Ville, which housed both the town hall and the police station, screeched left on the rue Vauban, and shot out the narrow, twisting road to Carsan. The death of the dog was a new and disturbing element. If its death could be traced directly to eating the bread, the whole texture of the emerging picture would be changed. It would no longer be a question of mild food poisoning with a brief illness, a quick recovery, and a happy prognosis. Up until this moment there had not been too much to be disturbed about, except the enormous number of patients. There were hundreds of cases of this sort in medical history, at church picnics, sporting events, holiday camps, where a temporary but vague element causes widespread but not serious damage.

The theory that M. Briand's bread was the cause of all this

was still not proven, and it was necessary not to jump to conclusions in spite of persuasive evidence. And if it were this bread, what would be the poison in it? No information had been circulated at this time about the illnesses in Connaux, or Bagnols-sur-Cèze, or the other towns, even among the doctors. In the cases involving the bread of M. Jaussent, no doctor in the village had been summoned, and both Dr. Gabbai and Dr. Vieu were ignorant at this time about the flurry that took place several days before. Most important, if M. Mison's case turned out to be as serious as his wife indicated over the phone, it was urgent to find out the exact source of the poison: The flour? The salt? The water? The yeast? The symptoms, though not too many had presented themselves to the overworked doctors at this time, did not seem to fit into any classical pattern. There was not enough of a distinctive clinical syndrome to permit exact and specific treatment. If M. Mison's case, in turning serious, foreshadowed other similar cases, the exact identification of the poison would become urgent.

Food poisoning took many forms. Chemical contaminants, such as heavy metals, fluorides, and others, were common. Toxins, increased by bacterial growth and a wide spectrum of organic substances that occur in natural foods, were other factors to be considered. The choices faced by Dr. Gabbai, if the outbreak suddenly turned serious, were confusing and numerous, especially without any clear-cut clinical symptoms to point the way to the discovery of the poison. Even typhoid, shigellosis, streptococcal pharyngitis, diphtheria, brucellosis, infectious hepatitis, and other diseases were often food-borne, although not necessarily classed as food poisoning. It was even necessary to consider epidemic nausea and vomiting arising from viruses.

As he drove into the farmyard of the Mison *domaine*, Dr. Gabbai realized the limitations he faced in the diagnosis of this strange problem, which was now becoming overwhelming.

Mme. Mison met him at the door. She was haggard and distraught. "It began shortly after your visit earlier," she said. "He was quiet for some time—then suddenly, without any warning, he jumped up out of bed and tried to run away from the house. He ran out into the yard like a wild man. Then he burst back in, dropped down on the bed again, and rolled back and forth. He was twisting and writhing—it was terrible. Then he shrieked in complete terror and huddled under his blankets, throwing them off, pulling them back up again, claiming he was either freezing or burning up. Right now he is mute. He is barely breathing. Please help us, Doctor. Please."

Dr. Gabbai went immediately to the bedside. Quickly he made his examination. The pupils were widely dilated. Temperature, subnormal. Pulse, slow and barely discernible. Respiration, labored and difficult. Sweating profusely. Blood pressure, far below normal. Extremities, cold. It was obvious that M. Mison was a desperately ill man on the verge of a cardiovascular collapse. Dr. Gabbai went immediately to the phone and called the hospital at Nîmes, nearly an hour away.

"There is nothing we can do here," he explained to Mme. Mison. "At the hospital they'll do all they can for your husband. Everything."

It took over an hour for the ambulance to arrive. During that time Dr. Gabbai fought to stay awake, tend his patient, and comfort the distraught Mme. Mison. He also had time to think about the phantom he was trying to fight.

The diagnosis was extremely difficult. Nearly every food poisoning brought on the same initial symptoms: abdominal pain, diarrhea, vomiting. But here was a case, and the others too in lesser form, with a whole new complex of clinical symptoms which failed to fit any set pattern. In salmonella gastroenteritis, for instance, there was nearly always a fever, but here the temperature was nearly always subnormal. In addition, the extreme dilation of the pupils and the strange psychical outbreak revealed in M. Mison's case did not seem to fit into any conventional food-poisoning pattern. Botulism was another possibility, but in none of the cases were the conventional symptoms for this condition prevalent to any degree: sudden hoarseness, constipation, cranial nerve paralysis. Staphylococcal food poisoning did cause lowered temperature and blood pressure, but support of this diagnosis would have to wait for further tests.

It was a question now of fighting a phantom whose name and identity were not known. Until they were known, only the most superficial treatment could be given, treatment for symptoms rather than causes. Until this case there had been no real emergency situation, since most of the patients appeared to be on the mend after a light touch of abdominal trouble. There had been a few odd symptoms, it was true, but they, too, had seemed to be on the verge of disappearing.

It was also possible that M. Mison was not suffering from the suspected bread but from another disease, which would require laboratory tests and careful hospital analysis. The most fearsome possibility stayed in the back of Dr. Gabbai's mind as a result of what Mme. Mison told him about over the phone: the death of the dog shortly after eating the suspected bread.

As casually as possible, to try to avoid disturbing her, he confirmed the incident with Mme. Mison as they waited. It was vital to correlate the information, and every small clue would help. The dog had eaten exclusively the bread bought from M. Briand that afternoon. It had not yet had its regular food. It had broken out in a most grotesque and horrifying fit—most unnatural and terrifying.

The headlights of the ambulance shined through the kitchen door, and it skidded to a stop just outside. Gently and with care, M. Mison was carried out, just as the first streaks of dawn were appearing in the sky over Mont Ventoux in the distance. Mme. Mison entered the ambulance beside her husband, and nodded her head in silent prayer. Dr. Gabbai watched them leave, and suddenly became aware of the overwhelming exhaustion that enveloped him. But time was pressing hard now, and he climbed into the car to drive back to the village. Winding down the hill from Carsan, he drove directly into the rising sun, which accented the burning in his eyes. He had had no sleep during the night, and only a little the night before. Perhaps he was overconcerned about the spread of the sickness. Perhaps the worst was over. But it was no time to take chances.

He drove directly to the home of Mayor Hebrard and pounded on the door until the mayor opened it, sleepily, to let him in.

"We're facing a severe crisis," he told the mayor. "M. Mison is seriously ill, and I have strong doubts about his survival. All the evidence points to the suspected bread. His dog died from eating it. We must call together both Dr. Vieu and Dr. Channac, if he's well enough now to help us. This may be more serious than we have thought."

Within half an hour the two other doctors had arrived. Dr.

Gabbai gave them the details of M. Mison's case and then learned that neither of the other two doctors had themselves been to bed the night before. Their phones had been continually ringing all night long. It was impossible to tell how many people without phones of their own would have been calling if it had been possible. The symptoms of the patients were exactly the same as those Dr. Gabbai had observed. And after the temporary improvement of the previous day, several patients now appeared more seriously ill.

The total number of cases among the doctors had now risen to over 280. Mme. Charpail's pseudo-epileptic fit now seemed to fit into the pattern, because the other two doctors reported similar reactions among their patients. Most disturbing was a confirming report from Dr. Vieu about the effect of the unknown poison on animals. Dr. Vieu had arrived at the home of Joseph Moulin to find the entire family and the work crew suffering from the same symptoms that had now become *classiques* at Pont-Saint-Esprit. Young Joseph Moulin was suffering the most—aching joints, alternate shivering and burning, low blood pressure, slow pulse, all the rest. His father was also in bad condition, and although Mme. Moulin suffered less than the others, she was by no means lightly ill. But, Dr. Vieu had learned, every animal on the Moulin farm that had eaten the bread was now dead—a fact that, joined with the evidence of the death of the Mison dog, almost unmistakably pinpointed the source of the trouble as the Briand bread and also foreshadowed far more serious consequences than the preliminary findings had indicated.

The tracing of the source of the poison was, of course, urgent, and both Dr. Vieu and Dr. Gabbai had instructed their patients to hold on to not only the remains of the bread that had been eaten but also the bodies of the animals who had been stricken so suddenly and violently. *Le médecin-chef* of the département du Gard, along with the prefect of Nîmes and the *gendarmerie*, would be arriving within hours from Nîmes. In the meantime the doctors would be treating the symptoms as best they could, until the samples of the food and the corpses of the animals could be rushed to the police scientific laboratories in Marseilles. Dr. Gabbai would keep in constant touch with the medical authorities at the hospital in Nîmes regarding the case of Félix Mison. His instinct and experience told him that it would be fortunate if M. Mison lasted twenty-four hours. A meeting at the Town Hall—*La Mairie*—was scheduled for eight that evening, after the doctors had had a chance to cover as many patients as possible during the day. As far as sleep was concerned, for the doctors that would be out of the question. Dr. Vieu, his own wife and family in bed and ill from the poisoning, had barely had time during the night to follow their progress. So great was the tide of calls pouring into the telephones of all three doctors that there were stretches of hours when they had to remain unanswered. Dr. Channac, still ill himself, painfully planned to continue his rounds as usual.

On Sunday morning, August 19, shortly after the doctors had had their meeting with Mayor Hebrard, Mlle. Wullschleger rose to dress for early mass at the Église Saint-Saturnin. She was sharply disturbed by the report, sent to her by messenger at the office, that her employer, M. Delacquis, was unable to return to the office because of illness. He had looked so weak, so pained, when he left the office just before noon on Saturday, that her heart had gone out to him. She would, she now determined, light a candle for him that morning at the church. Like many of the other citizens of the village she was still unaware of the extent of the outbreak, whatever it was. The doctors and the mayor had carefully avoided passing the word around in order not to spread any kind of panic among the populace. The problem of treating an unknown enemy was massive enough, without having to deal with hysteria.

When she arrived outside the church, she saw the clusters of people that had gathered to talk, and they talked only of the strange disease sweeping the town.

"*Mon Dieux*," one parishioner said to her as she arrived for the 8:30 mass. "Do you realize what has happened? Everybody in the village is sick. They say it comes from the bread of M. Briand."

"No," said another, "it comes from the water. Something has gone wrong with the water supply."

"It's the heat," said a third. "*Le soleil brule tous les temps. C'est terrible!*"

"The animals," a farmer from nearby added. "All the animals are dying. None of them in the region will live another day!"

Mlle. Wullschleger was shocked, but she did not immediately associate the sickness of M. Delacquis with the rumors now sweeping the town. His problem, according to the messenger, was fish, not bread. And she was sure he would be well and able to work by Monday.

She went into the ancient cathedral, through the weathered, massive door that had greeted the parishioners since 1475, went to a pew in the rear of the church, and kneeled in prayer. Beside her seat, on a stone pillar, was inscribed the Lord's Prayer as translated into the Provençal dialect by Frédéric Mistral:

O NOSTE PAIRE
QUE SIES CEU
TOUN NOUM SE SANTIFQUE!
TOUN REGNE NOUS AVENGUE!
ADAVAU TA VOULANTA SE FAGUE
COUME ADAMOUNT!

She read the words as music came forth from the organ, and they gave her comfort. She loved the saints, whose figures appeared in niches along the sides of the church, but she liked to pray directly to God, and she did. The church itself had remained there in the village for centuries and was a symbol of strength in the face of historical adversity. It had been rebuilt and reborn many times, through the ravages of time and the inhumanities of man. The people of Pont-Saint-Esprit were equally strong and tenacious, characteristics they would need if tragedy struck the town once again. She noticed also that there were many gaps in the congregation that morning—many more than usual. She looked up to the statue of St. Saturnin, serene in his niche near the altar, and drew further comfort from his countenance.

Also in the church that morning was Francine, who lighted a candle for her sister and prayed that the arm of the Virgin's statue would not symbolize another major tragedy for the town. Although she had forced the incident out of her mind, it returned in full force as she began to hear the stories circulating in the streets that Sunday morning. Worse was the condition of her sister, Mme. Charpail, who seemed to be sinking into a dark and distressing state with most mysterious symptoms. She would rise in the morning, go to the kitchen table in her mother's house, and sit vacantly staring down at the table for hours. Although her physical symptoms seemed to lessen, she would stay seated at the table, neither looking at, nor responding to, any of her family. When her nine-month-old baby was held in front of her, she would turn away from it or stare at it vacantly without recognition. If a glass of water or a piece of food was put in her hands, she would let it fall on the table or the floor. The prescribed medicines were useless, though at times her mother was able to force her to drink a cup of milk or sip an *infusion* of thyme, an ancient French remedy, popular in the Midi, which was made by pouring boiling water over leaves of thyme.

Francine prayed devoutly for her sister, as she did for the others in the village who were suffering and apparently facing a growing tragedy whose boundaries were nowhere in sight.

The only good news passed around after the mass that Sunday morning was that many people were apparently beginning to feel much stronger and better. In fact, one strange thing was that they were not only recovering but seemed to be experiencing an irresistible elation, their sense of well-being suddenly soaring to new and unprecedented heights, as if all their cares had been lifted and their problems dissolved. A sense of exaggerated fraternity had become apparent in some of the least likely people, who only a day before had been ill. One man, known for his rancor and disagreeable attitude, had embraced a former enemy on the streets and had suggested that old enmities be buried forever. Another, a man who had never been known to smile in the memory of most of the townspeople, had beamed and spoken with people to whom he had not spoken in years.

Another general observation seemed to emerge from the congregation after the services that day. Some of the people had noticed that since their brief illness they were infused with a force and energy they had never experienced before.

"You know," said a middle-aged lady to Mlle. Wullschleger as they were leaving the church, "I think this illness—whatever it is—has done me a lot of good. I've never had so much energy in my life. I know I haven't been able to sleep at all since Thursday evening, but I haven't been tired in the least. Last night I got up after trying to get to sleep for nearly an hour. I took out some sewing, thinking it would make me sleepy. I worked and I worked—and must have finished up more sewing than I could do in three days' time. I thought I would be so tired this morning that I would sleep all through the mass. But nothing like that happened. Right now I'm as wide awake as I've ever been, and I've never felt better."

As the woman talked, Mlle. Wullschleger could not help but notice that the woman's eyes had an abnormal luster and brilliance, that she was talking much faster than was her habit, and that she seemed to be inclined to go on talking forever. It was not the conversation of a person in robust health; it was more the strained, forced frenzy of a person bordering on hysteria.

After mumbling a polite *au revoir*, she left the still-talking woman, walked along the rue de la Paroisse in front of the church, then moved toward the stairs between the Église Saint-Saturnin and the twelfth-century Église Saint-Pierre. It was an empty but magnificent structure, which was never rebuilt after it had been pillaged during the French Revolution. From the terrace she could see the Rhône swirling southward, and the endless arches of the bridge that gave the village its name. From where she stood, the ghosts of history seemed to surround her on all sides. Not only had the Romans, the soldiers of the Wars of Religion, and the popes and antipopes been there, but the knights of three major Crusades had also marched through and stayed in the town on their way to the Holy Land. Even the presence of the English during the Hundred Years' War could be felt.

But this was the year of 1951, not the dark Middle Ages, and here was the possibility of a plague—and that was the accurate word, if what the villagers were saying was true—a plague as terrifying as those that had swept the village in medieval times. And what of modern science and medicine? From all reports bruited about after mass that morning, they had no effect whatever on those who were treated. And what about the diagnosis of the malady? None of the doctors had been able to give a clue. Yet people were suffering—no one knew exactly how many at this time—or becoming strangely hysterical in some form of euphoria that was totally meaningless and unsupported by objective reasons.

She left the plaza between the two churches and made her way back through the rue des Anciennes Prisons, toward the place de la République. Everywhere, groups of people, talking and gesticulating excitedly, were gathered in the narrow streets. Some refused to believe it was serious. Others predicted the end of the village, the country, the world.

Those among the townspeople who took the affair lightly were the most justified on that Sunday, because the actual confirmation of any serious reactions had not reached the populace yet, nor had the death of any animals been noted except by rumor. Only the doctors knew the actual extent of the sickness, and they continued to keep as silent as was possible about any serious future consequences. In spite of the buzzing conversations, there was a balance of optimism throughout the town, and the prevailing thought was that all would be over as the new week began.

The *boules* players were gathered as usual, and the sidewalk tables at the cafés along the Boulevard Gambetta were as full as usual on a Sunday noon. Whether it was at the Bar du Midi, the Café de Commerce, the Bar de l'Univers, the Rich Bar, or the bar where the club called La Boule Philosophie collected, the drinks were nearly all the same, the selection being limited to the popular *pastis*. The choice of *pastis* was multiple: Ricard, Pernod 45, Pastis 51, or other less famous brands. It would be ordered in many forms, whether with plain water, or in the form of a *tomate* (*pastis* with *sirop de grenadine*), a *péroquet* (*pastis* with *sirop de menthe*), or other mixtures, including *sirop d'Orgeat Fantasie*. In 1951 Scotch had not yet moved in to challenge Provence's favorite apéritif. But whatever those at the sidewalk cafés were drinking, their talk was of the sickness gripping the town, either scoffing at it or despairing of it.

Mlle. Wullschleger passed some of the cafés on her way to the house of her niece and her husband, a young married couple of the village. They were in mourning on this day because the husband's mother had died, and relatives were coming from as far away as Nîmes for the services to be held that afternoon. The death was a natural one, of old age, and had nothing whatever to do with the illness that was engulfing the town, but hearing in advance of the trouble, the relatives from out of town brought their own bread with them.

The lunch that Sunday was one of mourning, the men in their

hot, black suits and shoes; the women in equally heavy black dresses. Mlle. Wullschleger's niece, serving apricot tarts after the luncheon, noted with bitter irony that the tarts had actually saved them from the scourge in the town. She had gone, she explained, to Grande Rue to buy the pastry and bread for the weekend. Her regular *boulanger* was M. Briand, but out of impulse she had gone to a competitor's shop for the pastry and did not dare go then to buy the bread from M. Briand in the fear that he would notice the pastry and feel that she was disloyal. By this fortuitous stroke of embarrassment she and her family had been saved from further tragedy striking the household.

At the luncheon Mlle. Wullschleger could not keep her thoughts from wandering back to the pitiful figure of M. Delacquis as he left the office on his bicycle the previous day. With phones and transportation scarce it was impossible to receive further news of his condition at the moment. There was, it seemed, sadness everywhere in the village.

After he had thrown himself on the bed on Saturday afternoon, M. Delacquis felt too weak even to lift his head. The room would alternately spin and stop, then suddenly enlarge to enormous proportions before it would equally as suddenly shrink until he thought it would squeeze him to death. He closed his eyes, but could not sleep. As he did, visions of enormous flowers blossomed behind his closed eyelids. The flowers were not as if he were imagining them, but as if they were actually there in front of him. Yet he knew they were not real. The colors were the most vivid he had ever seen, blinding in their brilliance. When he opened his eyes again, he discovered that he had been undressed and was under the covers. He was sweating profusely, yet he was shivering at the same time. He looked at the window and saw that it, too, was enlarging in front of his eyes, encompassing the entire sky with its size until it shrank down again to an infinitely narrow slit. He seemed to have no relationship to time itself and was not aware of what day it was now or of what the others in the household were doing. Then, as suddenly as he felt ill and dizzy and was seized with *ivresse*, he would be flooded with a feeling of total ecstasy, of a beatitude he had never experienced. He yearned for a pencil and paper to write down a series of glorious insights about the universe that came into his consciousness, then disappeared as quickly. But he was too weak to move, and had no desire to call out for assistance.

In spite of the wild and irrational visions and colors that swept before him, the basic core of his consciousness remained rational. He was aware that what was happening was not real, yet what he saw and envisaged had all the attributes of total reality. He knew also that he would fade from consciousness, and was certain that was what had happened when he had been undressed and placed under the covers. He would find moments to worry and fret about the unfinished work at the office, and then when the tides of exhilaration came over him, when the mysterious sense of rapturous benignity swept through him, he felt no concern, no worry, but only the glory of a universe whose meaning he seemed to be seizing for the first time. He could hear vague sounds, vague voices outside the room, and he was conscious that several times Mme. Testevin entered, sometimes with Mme. Lamacchir. He was aware that they were changing his sheets, which were drenched with perspiration, softly wiping his forehead, then disappearing quietly out into the hallway. He was aware of them, but could not seem to communicate with them.

What M. Delacquis did not know, when Saturday evening came, was that the only people in the household able to be on their feet were M. and Mme. Lamacchir, who had eaten the bread they had brought with them, and Mme. Testevin. The latter, who had eaten only a piece of bread "no bigger than her little finger," was ill, too, but managed to be up and help with the others by sheer force of will and the fact that she had eaten so lightly.

Both Emile and M. Testevin had come in early from the vineyards, exhausted and dizzy. By supper time each had gone to bed, M. Testevin in the large room over the dining room, Emile in his quarters in the farm building adjoining the main villa. Mme. Dezeuzes, returning from the village just before supper time, excused herself from the others and retired to her room.

M. Testevin already suffered from a weak liver and was convinced, along with the others, that his suffering resulted from the trout. After he got into bed, he told Mme. Testevin that when he moved or tried to sit up, his head spun. Emile's complaints were the same. He stated that he felt as if he were very drunk, that the room was going around crazily, and that he was sure he would be all right in the morning. No one in the house yet associated their problems with the bread, and none of the news that was beginning to circulate along Grande Rue had reached La Villette by Saturday evening.

All through Saturday night and into the early hours of Sunday morning no one in the household was able to sleep, in spite of overwhelming exhaustion alternating with periods of exaggerated energy. Mme. Testevin finally dozed off toward morning, after having made many trips to the kitchen during the night to make endless cups of steaming lime-flower tea, known as *tilleul*. This was another common remedy in the Midi, a common practice for soothing and calming patients, as well as for scenting a baby's bath.

At six on Sunday morning Mme. Testevin woke from her catnap with a start. Strange sounds were coming from the courtyard, and she ran to the window to look out. Emile was lying naked in the middle of the yard near the stone washing well, writhing in agony. She swiftly ran downstairs and reached his side as the Lamacchirs, also hearing the sounds, rushed to help her.

The three of them helped him into the dining room, arranged a cot for him there, and tried to calm him down. By now M. Testevin was roused, and although still weak, he came down the stairs to see if he could help. The others pleaded with him to return to bed, but he insisted that he was fully recovered, and that he must immediately go into town to get the doctor. Before the others could stop him, he was out in the courtyard and mounting his bicycle. He moved off, uncertainly, through the courtyard, moving behind the stone wall and out of sight of the dining room window, from where the others were watching. They did not see him as the bicycle began wobbling crazily back and forth across the road until it shot out from under him and he sprawled across the road just as M. Delacquis had done the afternoon before. He managed to get to his feet and push the bicycle along the stone wall, still out of sight of the others, until he reached the end of the long farm building. There he climbed unsteadily into the truck and drove off down the road toward the village and the office of Dr. Gabbai.

FOUR

AFTER THE DAWN meeting with Mayor Hebrard, Dr. Gabbai drove to his home. He arrived there shortly after six, painfully aware that he would get no sleep this day. At his office window, where he tried to collect his thoughts and organize the day in the face of the disorganized chaos that was shaping up all over the village, he noticed the truck of M. Testevin making its uncertain way down the route de Bagnols toward his house. He watched in astonishment as M. Testevin pulled up by the curb, climbed out of the truck, then began crawling on his hands and knees toward the doorway. The doctor's first thought was that he was drunk. He opened the front door just as M. Testevin was climbing up the steps, still on his hands and knees.

M. Testevin blurted out the story: Everyone except the two visitors at La Villette was ill; Emile was in very bad condition. M. Testevin didn't care about himself, but the others. . . .

Dr. Gabbai, a friend of the Testevins for many years, knew that M. Testevin was a sober man, and a diligent one. He examined him minutely at the office, noting that in spite of his illness, M. Testevin was talking in a most euphoric way. He seemed to be on a cloud of unalloyed exaltation, while at the same time an objective examination revealed the same nagging symptoms plaguing all his patients in the past few days. The temperature, as expected, was subnormal, the pupils widely enlarged, the pulse slow, the blood pressure low. Along with many other patients now, M. Testevin also had a sharp and biting form of heartburn that would not respond to any usual ameliorative. When M. Testevin said that he had not slept for two nights in a row, and that he had moments when he felt the strength of ten men, interspersed with moments of deep depression, labored breathing, and thoughts that he was surely going to die, Dr. Gabbai nodded in affirmation, because these symptoms were now being noted almost universally among the patients.

The examination over, the doctor now faced the moment that was becoming more frustrating by the hour: What to prescribe? No word could be expected yet from the police laboratory in Marseilles; the symptoms were rare and not clearly recognizable. Each of the doctors had theories, but these could not be confirmed without the laboratory tests, and at this stage of the progress of the epidemic it could only be guess work.

In between the frenzied visits to patients Dr. Gabbai was painstakingly preparing a chart of symptoms, but there was little time to correlate it now. New symptoms seemed to be appearing daily.

With considerable difficulty, for M. Testevin was a large man, Dr. Gabbai helped him into his own car and left the truck to be taken care of later. He stopped at a pharmacy for some additional medicine in the hope of treating the symptoms before driving out to La Villette. One pharmacy—that of M. Charrière—bore an ominous sign on the door: FERMÉE POUR CAUSE DE MALADIE.

The pharmacists, as well as the physicians, were so deluged with clients that their shops were filled day and night. In France the pharmacist often assumes the role of a doctor for the lighter afflictions of those in the village, and the current disturbing illness was no exception. Each day, in the regional paper from Marseilles or from Montpellier, a doctor and a pharmacist were customarily listed under the village name for emergency duty during the night. The notices continued to appear at this time as usual. But all the doctors and the pharmacists—except those who were stricken badly themselves—were on call all day and all night, simply because of the overwhelming pressure of the circumstances. Staggering the work load was out of the question.

On the way back to La Villette, M. Testevin remained in his state of *euphorie béate,* despite his other symptoms. He now revealed also a marked increase in the flow of saliva.

At La Villette only Mme. Testevin and the guests from Toulon were out of bed. They helped the doctor remove M. Testevin from the car and gingerly guided him up the narrow staircase to his room.

Dr. Gabbai began his examinations of the others. Emile, on the cot in the dining room, was writhing in pain and sweating profusely. With the sweating was a rancid odor, an odd mixture of smells, as if it were of dead mice and stale urine. The doctor had noticed this on his visit to M. Mison—was this another symptom to be added now to the mélange? He noted convulsive contractions of the muscles, a symptom of tetanus, or epilepsy, or meningitis—or what?

Emile's eyes, their pupils swollen in size, looked at him pleadingly. He had not slept for two days and nights; like the others his exhaustion was great. He moved from weakness to strength in alternating cycles, however, and his strength, when it came, was like that of a drunkard: enormous and uncontrolled. The doctor's problem was that nothing administered seemed to help, even symptomatically. Barbiturates in extremely strong doses were useless to combat the growing insomnia. Morphine, chloral hydrates, or the hypnotic drugs seemed to be equally ineffective. Furthermore, in 1951, postwar scarcities in France were still in effect. Dimly hopeful that this case might be an exception, he prescribed a sedative and then went up to the room of Mme. Dezeuzes.

She was on the bed and crying. She, like the others, had not been able to sleep. Her physical symptoms were close to those of the others. Although her digestive troubles had subsided, her psychological depression was great and unrelenting. She was helpless when she tried to get up to assist Mme. Testevin, and her sense of guilt about this assumed an exaggerated form, which increased her depression. Unlike the others, her periods of euphoria were brief, even though intense. After prescribing for her, Dr. Gabbai moved on to the room of M. Delacquis.

He was on his bed, with a tablet on his knees and a pencil in his hand, writing. He had already filled one pad and was beginning his second. Although his mind seemed clear and his handwriting steady, he seemed distant and unrelated to his surroundings. Like the others, he was sweating, so that even now his sheets, which had been changed within the hour, were soaking wet. Again, the odor of dead mice, strong and overbearing. Again, the low blood pressure, the slow pulse, the wide pupils. In addition to the *mydriase*—the large pupils—Dr. Gabbai noted a new symptom for the first time. The artery serving his left eye was swollen and dangerously pathological; it showed up clearly as the doctor looked at the retina through the ophthalmoscope. The room was sweltering with the heat of the Provençal August, yet the doctor noticed that M. Delacquis was under three blankets and still shivering with cold as the sweat poured off him. His extremities were frigid, and yet he seemed to be burning up at the same time. After administering a sedative, the doctor suggested to M. Delacquis that he should stop writing on the tablet and rest. The suggestion was politely but firmly refused.

Down in the kitchen the doctor asked Mme. Testevin if she could get further help to take care of the four *malades* who were depending so much on her. She told him that Mme. Lamacchir was insisting that she stay on to help and that the Mlles. Rigaud, two sisters who lived in a neighboring farmhouse, had volunteered to help in the mornings. Mme. Testevin herself had not slept since the trouble began, but her digestive upset seemed to have cleared up and her strength was holding up well, almost too well, in the face of the lack of sleep. The doctor tried to persuade her to get some rest. He knew she would keep the others as comfortable as possible and let him know if any crisis occurred among the four patients scattered through the rooms of the villa.

"I would give every stone of the house," she told the doctor, "if I could get them well."

The doctor, sagging more than ever with his own exhaustion, patted her on the shoulder and went out to the courtyard and his car.

Sunday was always a welcome day at the home of M. and Mme. Eynard, for their dental office was crowded the other six days of the week from early morning until eight in the evening. As the only dentists in the surrounding area, their work schedule allowed little time for recreation, although they were enthusiastic skiers and campers. They looked forward to the time when the postwar years would gradually bring more professional men into the area, so that their time for leisure would be more available.

This Sunday, August 19, brought none of the joy of relief they usually felt. The talk and the rumors circulating around the village were far too disquieting, and the mystery seemed to be growing rather than receding. In midmorning someone knocked on the door of their home on the Boulevard Gambetta. It was one of their patients, an elderly woman, who told them that a friend of theirs who lived on the place de l'Hôtel de Ville had asked her to let them know that he was very ill, living alone, and unable to cope with the sudden situation. He was an engineer of whom the Eynards were very fond, a technician at the nearby glass factory. M. Eynard lost no time following the woman out of the door and hastening toward the house where his friend was rooming.

Passing Grande Rue, M. Eynard noted the exceptional number of people in the streets, all of them talking with an abnormal intensity.

"What is it, *cher Docteur?*" a man from one of the groups asked him as he was passing. "Is it what they say—does it come from the drinking water? Or from the salt? Or the meat?"

M. Eynard, who had already talked to all three of his medical colleagues, was at a loss as to what to reply. None of the symptoms, he had been told, added up to a clear manifestation of any known current disease.

"I'm afraid we will have to await the tests from Marseilles," he told the man.

"But how long, *Docteur?* How long must we wait? So many people are suffering!"

Like every other professional man in the village, M. Eynard devoutly wished that he were able to answer the question. Not since the Middle Ages had an unknown and mysterious malady ranged throughout the village, and the atmosphere was already charged with that sort of feeling. There was no panic yet; the rumors were conflicting and served to neutralize each other, so that even the strong suspicion that the source could be traced to the bread of M. Briand remained on the same level as the other rumors. No official public announcement had yet been made; that would wait until after the meeting. And perhaps, if M. Mison survived, and the symptoms subsided generally, no pronouncement would be necessary. Nothing was moving in terms of rational prediction; the unexpected was becoming routine. Not knowing the source of the trouble exactly, each villager seemed to be developing his own theories.

At the bedside of his engineer friend M. Eynard listened to his story. All Saturday night he had been unable to sleep. He had risen at about three and tried to read, but the pages danced in front of his eyes. Then a compulsion to walk came over him, even though he felt weak and dizzy. He dressed and went out into the narrow streets of the village. The shadows and the darkness seemed ominous to him at first. He walked down along the Rhône all the while trying to resist what he felt was a ridiculous impulse to walk. He found himself crossing the entire length of the bridge, then turning and coming back into town, a round trip of over two miles. He could not understand his own wakefulness, or his passionate desire to walk.

Reaching the Boulevard Gambetta, he was shocked to find that he was not the only one in the village who could not sleep. Several groups of people were gathered there, standing in clusters and talking ceaselessly. Although he was new to the village, he was welcomed cordially, as if a sudden fraternity had sprung up among the sleepless. They were talking about the sickness spreading over the village, but their talk was predominantly in a most light and frivolous manner. Many were laughing and joking about it; no one felt any desire to go back to bed. One told of a friend of his who had been stricken by the malady and had thrown up four litres of clear gastric fluid; this was found to be most amusing. The ripples of laughter from the groups were forced, high pitched, and eerie. The whole scene, in the darkness of the early morning hours, was most unnatural. The people were standing in ghostly silhouette under the plane trees, standing as if this were full daylight at the market place. Others were walking at random, very quickly, along the streets and *allées*, without destination, speaking to no one.

He eventually excused himself from the group, returned to his room, and lay down on the bed in a futile attempt to get to sleep.

It was impossible. His mind kept inexplicably turning to the thought of potatoes, potatoes of every size and shape. He was amused at this thought at first—why should he be thinking of potatoes in the middle of the night, or rather just before dawn? The whole idea was ludicrous, and he found himself laughing out loud about it. But after half an hour had gone by, and he found he simply could not get the thought of potatoes out of his mind, he became desperately anxious about it. It now became a challenge to rid himself of this compulsion, to convince himself of the ridiculous drain of energy this involved.

It was only in the early morning, when he heard the cars and traffic in the street, that the thought of potatoes slowly faded from his mind.

But now his stream of consciousness was overwhelmed by another idea, an idea that became so overpowering he actually felt he was losing his mind: Every time a car or a truck rumbled by in the street below, he was utterly and absolutely convinced that the house around him was going to come tumbling down. It was not a question of this being a remote possibility; he was *sure* it would happen. He would hear an automobile in the distance. His muscles would tighten. He would clench his teeth almost automatically. Then the sound of the motor would grow louder as the car approached. He would throw his arms over his head and wait for the ripping sound of falling timbers and the crash of the stones from the house. When nothing would happen, he would steel himself again, waiting for the next car to come along.

He explained to M. Eynard that he had not felt sick enough to call a doctor, and he knew how busy they were. He was feeling stronger now, and some of his feelings about the house collapsing around him were fading.

M. Eynard listened and found himself wondering if the sickness was perhaps going to strike him and his family, too. They had escaped any trouble up to now, but the pattern of the disease—whatever it was—was so unpredictable that it spread fear rapidly throughout the town. He arranged to bring food and wine to his friend and invited him to come to the Eynard house at any time of night or day. Meanwhile, they would visit him regularly and see that care was taken of him. If the symptoms became worse, Eynard would bring the doctor. The engineer had stubbornly insisted he did not want a doctor at this time. M. Eynard took his leave as a truck rattled by in the street below.

"This time," said the engineer, "I feel no fear. Perhaps getting it off my chest to you has cured me!"

At home again the Eynards tried to make sense out of what was becoming a most alarming and confused situation. As dentists, they were professionally aware of many of the medical ailments of the human body, but they could not distinguish any sort of rationality in the puzzle.

"Francine's sister still doesn't seem to respond to anything," Mme. Eynard said, after her husband told her about his visit. "She sits there at the kitchen table and stares down at the floor. She won't touch her baby. They are all terribly upset. The only good thing I've heard is that M. Sauvet is feeling much better. He was so sick yesterday that his wife had almost given up hope."

"When this first happened," said M. Eynard, "I was sure it was a case of simple ptomaine poisoning. I never thought I'd find myself in the position of wishing that ptomaine poisoning would strike. But that would be a lot better than what we have now."

"All we need to know now," said Mme. Eynard with a weak smile, "is when is it going to strike us?"

All through the day on Sunday Dr. Gabbai kept in touch with the doctors at the hospital at Nîmes. The news concerning M. Mison was not good. Laboratory tests were inconclusive in attempting to find the cause of the condition, and he was failing fast. The doctors at Nîmes faced the same phantom as Dr. Gabbai. It was impossible to treat the disease without an exact knowledge of the cause. The laboratory tests of the bread at the police scientific laboratory would take time; it was impossible to rush them. Many exacting analytical steps were required. M. Mison was meanwhile receiving treatment for symptoms; it was all that could possibly be done under the circumstances.

One theory that was growing in the minds of the doctors, since the evidence pointed to the bread as a source, was a rare disease known as ergotism. It had reached plague proportions during the Middle Ages but had practically disappeared from the face of the earth in modern times. It was not until 1670 that ergot was identified as a parasitic mold growing on rye and wheat under extremely rare conditions. The disquieting thing about ergotism, if this were indeed the disease, is that there is no known cure, even in modern medicine.

When he returned from the Testevin farm, Dr. Gabbai's office was full, and his phone was ringing persistently. Generally, the digestive troubles were subsiding. In their place was the rising and persistent insomnia. Complaint after complaint over the inability to sleep came from the patients, both those in the office and those on the house calls. Some said they felt such an imminent and overwhelming premonition of death that they panicked during the night. Others complained about sweating so profusely that they had to change their clothes several times a day. The odor of dead mice and of stale urine from the sweat was constant, with the rancid pungency penetrating the household. The sweating was accompanied by an unquenchable thirst. Many felt an overwhelming compulsion to commit suicide.

Instead of being disquieted by their symptoms, many of the patients seemed irrationally pleased and elated with themselves and their condition. Their moods would alternate. Some of the patients talked at such a rapid rate that it was impossible for the doctor to understand them. They refused to be interrupted for the simple and basic questions the doctor had to ask. They talked of feeling a grand enlightenment, a sweeping feeling of beatitude and euphoria which only occasionally was broken by spells of anguish and depression. Some were seized by a vicious and agonizing form of heartburn, along with an icy coldness in the hands and feet. The low blood pressure, the subnormal temperatures, the enlarged pupils, continued to show up during the visits. Dr. Gabbai, a warm and sympathetic man, faced the frustration of fighting against the unknown; his sympathies and regard for his friends and patients were being strained to the breaking point by the lack of specific medical treatment to offer.

The meeting on Sunday night at the Hôtel de Ville did not begin until nine but continued until one o'clock Monday morning. Along with Mayor Hebrard were the entire Municipal Council, the chief medical officer of the Gard *département*, the three local doctors, the local police, the *gendarmes*, and representatives of the office of the public prosecutor at Nîmes. The meeting was grim and quiet. Since no deaths had occurred, there was hope that all would begin to improve within the next few days. As a precaution, however, experts would be summoned from the University of Montpellier's medical school and from the University of Marseilles. The *procureur de la République,* as the public prosecutor was known, and the *juge d'instruction,* the examining magistrate, would be called in to begin a thorough but quiet investigation in order to avoid unduly alarming the population. Meanwhile, Commissioner Sigaud, a detective of the Fourteenth Mobile Brigade, would begin an immediate inquiry into the facts of the case. More samples of the bread would be taken and rushed to the police laboratories at Marseilles, along with the cadavers of the Moulin and Mison animals; the results of the initial tests would be pressed with the utmost haste. Some were grumbling that there were too many delays in the investigation.

The atmosphere was taut, but there was no panic at the meeting. Only the exhaustion of the physicians, and now of the mayor, indicated the seriousness of the situation. There was still hope that on Monday the tide would subside. There had been meetings like this before in Pont-Saint-Esprit, in the deep past of the Middle Ages, when cholera or the bubonic plague had struck. These had been meetings of panic and terror, when people dropped in the streets and doctors collapsed at the bedsides of their patients. The scene and the backdrop were the same in August of 1951, but now there was modern science with all its available resources to combat the disease. It would only be a matter of time until the laboratory tests would be completed, the cause determined, and the disease conquered. Perhaps, after it was all over, the only inconvenience would prove to be the closing of the bakeries and the eating of *biscottes*—the hard, packaged rusks in the shape of bread slices—which, of course, could never substitute for the bread by which the villagers lived.

At one o'clock on Monday morning, when the meeting broke up, Dr. Gabbai walked down the blackened Boulevard Gambetta to his home, only two blocks away. The shadows of the groups under the plane trees were there, the news of the meeting having accented the inquietude of the insomniacs. The state of nervous, elated excitement was still evident. He knew, without seeing in the dark, what many of their faces were like in this strange state of euphoria: a wan visage, a somewhat waxy tint to the skin, yet with the persistent expression of beatitude. Occasionally, a voice from one group would call in the distance to another. The whole aspect of the village seemed to be changing; daytime habits were becoming those of night. Rarely were the streets of the village occupied at night; even the cafés closed early by habit. Now it was different, as if the villagers were waiting for something vague and mysterious. But the anxiety was not major; it was a waiting, and for what, not even Dr. Gabbai knew.

Holding back any major anxiety on the part of the villagers was the fact that, while they knew and talked incessantly about the malady striking, and striking often, at least it did not kill. Time after time the phrase would come out among the restless, sleepless groups on Boulevard Gambetta: "*La peste frappe . . . la peste frappe souvent, mais il ne tue pas! Dieu merci!*" The plague strikes often, but thank God it doesn't kill!

In this many took comfort, because the shadow of *la peste*—the plague, as they were beginning to call it—could fall on anyone, anytime apparently. It seemed always to be a matter of who was to be next.

Dr. Gabbai had come to expect his phone to be ringing any time he entered his house. Returning from the meeting at the Hôtel de Ville in the darkness of Monday morning, he found no exception. It was now about 1:30 A.M. Automatically, he picked up the phone, answered it in a voice now becoming hoarse from constant consultations with his patients, twenty-four hours around the clock. It was Mme. Renée Carle, who helped her husband run their grocery on the rue Joliot Curie, an extension of the Grande Rue, a short distance away from the bakery of M. Briand.

"Forgive me, doctor, for calling you at this time of the morning," she said. "Please forgive me. But our daughter. She's just five you know. Marie-Joseph. It's frightening. It's terrible. I just can't describe it . . ."

Her voice trailed off in sobs.

Dr. Gabbai reached for his bag, which never left his side these days. "I'll be right over," he said.

He hung up the phone, and because the Carles were so near, decided to walk the few hundred feet, through the place de la République, to the Carle home. Other groups of the sleepless were there, standing outside the Café de la Bourse, although its windows were darkened and the chairs piled on the tables.

"Any more news, *Docteur?*" asked a sweltering, undershirted man from the group.

"None at the moment," said the doctor. "You should try to sleep."

"We do," said another. "We do try. *Mais c'est impossible!*"

"Have courage," said the doctor, and plunged into the blackness of the rue Joliot Curie.

Joseph Carle and his family lived above their grocery store in an ancient house now neatly restored and not far from the place de la Libération and the rue du 15 Août 1944. Mme. Carle let him in through the darkened front door of the store and led him along the rows of foodstuffs and up the inside stairway.

Dr. Gabbai had already made several calls on the Carle family, since everybody, including the *femme de ménage* was stricken to some degree. M. Carle was still bedridden but seemed to be improving, even though he had gone without sleep since Friday night. Massive doses of barbituates had failed to relieve him. As in many of the stricken households, the family had blamed the malady on bad meat. At the present stage M. Carle was listless but wakeful. Every time he tried to get up, dizziness would force him to lie down again. Confined to his room, he was desperate to be at the side of his daughter, but he fell to the floor every time he tried.

From the moment he entered the door, Dr. Gabbai could hear the shrieks of five-year-old Marie-Joseph. When he saw her, the sight was shocking even for a doctor of his long experience. Her entire body was shaking; her arms and legs were jerking in massive spasms; her fingers were clenched until they were white; her toes were bent under so rigidly that they could not be pried open. Her eyes were moving wildly in their sockets, and her contracting arm muscles gave her the appearance of a choral director leading a choir.

"Mama!" she was screaming. "Mama! The tigers! They are going to eat me! They are going to bite me!"

Her eyes would widen, then focus on the wall in front of her. "There!" she cried. "Right there! Beside the wall! Can't you see them? Mama, stop them from biting me!"

There was no question that she was seeing the tigers, which were as real as if they had been there. In another moment she was seeing serpents on the curtains. She was screaming and writhing to get away from them. Dr. Gabbai lost no time in administering a sedative intravenously and then methodically going about his examination. Mme. Carle stood by, in tears, stroking the forehead of the child, who was drenched in perspiration.

"Mama!" she screamed again. "Mama, I am going to die! There is blood dripping from the ceiling!"

The examination revealed an extreme state of cardiovascular collapse. The writhing and convulsions continued, and so did the hallucinations. While waiting for the results of the sedative, the doctor placed a towel over her eyes, which immediately changed the color of the tigers she saw, but did nothing to remove them. After fifteen minutes it was obvious that the sedative had no effect whatever.

"There is only one thing to do," said the doctor. "We must call in a specialist from Avignon. They have many specialists for children at the hospital there. They will do everything they can to help."

He moved wearily to the phone to call the hospital, but stopped momentarily to see M. Carle, who was propped up on his bed by his elbows.

"*Docteur*," he said. "I must have the curtains for the doorway with beads on them. You've got to help me get them. For the flies. The flies must have curtains with beads on them. Will you help me get them? For the flies. The flies have great need for curtains with beads on them. You understand? They need them. Curtains with beads on them . . ."

His head fell back on the square pillow and bolster, his words turning into meaningless mumbling.

Dr. Gabbai's exhausted mind began to doubt the sanity of the world itself. What new symptoms were these that were beginning to manifest themselves? Vivid hallucinations in a five-year-old child. Obsessional compulsion in her father, an *idée fixe* that had imposed itself forcefully on his mind.

He administered a sedative to the father, then went back to the child's room. As the doctor left, M. Carle turned his attention now to the window in his room. There were six panes in it, and he began counting them, aloud: One, two, three, four, five, six; one, two, three, four, five, six; one, two, three, four, five, six. He was not to stop counting them for nearly three weeks, day and night, without sleep.

In her room, Marie-Joseph had suddenly become calm. She was no longer confused and was wide awake and fully normal in appearance. Her blood pressure was improved. She remembered the tigers and the snakes clearly, and seemed to understand that even though she had actually seen them with her eyes in the room, they were not real. She could describe exactly what she saw, but she seemed to realize that they were illusory figures. "I guess it was like a wide-awake dream, Mama," she said.

It was hard to tell if her new calm came from the sedative or from a spontaneous recovery. The doctor was inclined to think the latter, for the child was far too wide-awake and alert to reflect the effect of a heavy sedative. But under these conditions, he decided to hold off calling the hospital at Avignon in the hope that the sudden recovery might hold. By now Mme. Carle was calmer too, and the doctor left her with instructions to call him at any time if a relapse should occur.

Although he longed desperately for sleep, he knew that the likelihood of it was next to impossible. He would make himself some strong coffee when he arrived home, and perhaps he would be able to take a nap in the chair in his office before the next call came. But even this devout hope was optimistic. As he opened the door, the phone was ringing, shattering the early morning darkness with its persistence. He dropped heavily onto his chair behind his desk and answered it. It was the Hôpital Gaston Domergue de Nîmes.

Félix Mison, the farmer from Carsan, was dead.

All during the days that the doctors of Pont-Saint-Esprit had been without sleep, no word concerning the sickness had appeared in the regional newspapers of Montpellier and Marseilles, the only two papers serving the region. The reasons were varied. The evidence of the extent of the plague—*la peste*—gathered slowly and erratically. In spite of the constant gossip in the streets and cafés, most of the villagers felt that the next day would bring better news. Even the doctors, noting a sharp decline in the severity of the symptoms after the second day, were inclined to think that the worst was over. As the evidence piled up, the authorities were anxious to prevent panic, and made no official pronouncements. The strange state of *euphorie béate* was also contagious to a degree, creating an atmosphere of lightheartedness that rode over the feelings of numerous families as they noted the marked improvement of their own *malades* at varying moments.

On Monday, August 20, only a few hours after Dr. Gabbai had received the news of M. Mison's death, the streets of the village came to life much as on any other day. The strain of the past few days had caused a tolerance for the news of someone being suddenly stricken, and those who did fall ill were now regarded merely as delayed fuses in a disturbing but undulating situation in which good news of apparent recovery seemed to match the bad news of disheartening setbacks. The undercurrent, the murmurs, though, continued. Friends of the Carle family brought to Grande Rue the story of Marie-Joseph's night, when she had seen tigers and watched blood drip from the ceiling. M. Sauvet, the *garagiste*, had a relapse and was making no progress whatever; he was still unable to get out of bed. Gossip regarding the conditions at La Villette were highly disturbing. Mme. Testevin, it was said, was exhausted from trying to take care of four patients. A procession of friends drove or walked to the farmhouse with gifts and offers to help. But this frequently served to make the situation there more disorganized. The nagging fear hanging over most of the households yet untouched still remained: Will we be next?

But all this was within tolerable limits of the villagers' endurance. They waited and hoped for better news to break.

Just where the first information came from is uncertain. Dr. Gabbai had not announced it, nor had the authorities. It happened sometime in midmorning. There were no details. The word seemed to strike Grande Rue, the cafés, the Boulevard Carnot, the Boulevard Gambetta, the shops, the houses, the vineyards, the ancient hospital, the public washing basins, the post office, the river front, at one single electrifying moment, as if the news were announced from the high tower of the cathedral to the tolling of bells for all to hear. It was not so announced, of course, but it might as well have been. It could be said in one sentence:

"*Le pain tue!*"

Up until this moment, Gallic resignation had held back real terror and panic; had served as a dam against pressures that had been inexorably building up, but seldom expressed outwardly. Now the single sentence was almost literally on every lip: "*The bread kills!*" For nearly three hundred families, a sword of Damocles seemed to be hoisted over the thresholds. A stillness and quiet descended, for the three words of the sentence were all that were needed to be said. Yes, it was M. Mison: a *gentil* man who was loved and respected all around the countryside. A man whose dog had died, in pain and convulsions, only a short while before.

Clusters of people gathered, by the fountains and in the streets. They were not talking excitedly now. The voices were hushed. "*Le pain tue!*" It was a whisper louder than any shout.

FIVE

Arriving back from the Ardèche, M. Briand found himself wondering, as he had during his visit to his children, why he felt no fatigue whatever after three sleepless nights. He was further concerned about his wife, who seemed to be alternately sick and well all during their weekend trip.

His daughter Yvonne was the first to give him the news, early on Monday morning.

"Every *boulangerie* in the village is closed, Papa," she said. "We've been ordered to shut down."

M. Briand was stunned.

"But why?" he said.

"There is much sickness in all the village," Yvonne said. "They think it is our bread that has done it."

"But that's impossible," Briand said. "How could it be our bread?"

The gray flour from the north came quickly to his mind, of course. But all the bakers had been forced to use it. How would his be different from the others?

"Both Dr. Gabbai and Dr. Vieu were here while you were

gone," Yvonne said. "They say that there cannot be any mistake. They are sure now."

Within the hour Dr. Gabbai came to visit.

"It seems your bread is making everyone ill," he said.

"It just can't be," said Briand. "I use only water and salt and yeast—exactly the same as the other bakers. The flour from the north has been gray—yes. But all of us have been using it."

"We are doing everything we can to find out," said the doctor. "Everything. But it is taking time."

"Is anyone seriously ill?" Briand asked.

"That's what I must tell you," said the doctor quietly. "M. Mison died this morning."

M. Briand sunk in his chair. He dropped his head in his hands. "What did I do wrong, Doctor? What did I do wrong?" The question turned over and over in his mind. He went back over all the details of his *fournées* during the past week. Was this the ultimate climax of the battle with the Union Meunière? But if so, why had it not happened before, and why hadn't the bread of the other bakers been involved? All the sick villagers had been traced to his bakery, and to his alone. And then there was M. Mison. M. Briand recalled Mison's visit to the shop vividly—the joking and the chiding because he had forgotten to make his delivery in Carsan that day. Now Mison was dead. Hundreds of others were sick. Including himself—and his wife, who was now forced to her bed. His daughter Yvonne had eaten only the *brioche* on that day. She was well. The theory of the doctors was even proved true within his own family. And what about his helper, Aimé Pradier? Briand was to learn soon that M. Pradier was desperately ill also.

Within a few hours, the *commissaires* from the public prosecutor's office in Nîmes arrived at M. Briand's door, and the full inquiry began.

The tidal wave of panic in the village, as it began, was an enormous swell rather than a crashing breaker. The feeling everywhere was one of being trapped, with nowhere to go, with nothing to do about it. Modern medicine seemed to do nothing. The theory that it was the bread was still not fully established. The feeling that it might be the water or a strange communicable disease of unknown origin persisted. Some quietly packed and went to visit relatives or friends in other villages, unable to stand what they called "the agonizing suspense." Others stayed on their farms. The shops were half empty. The doctors were seen in the streets, constantly crossing and recrossing each other's paths on their way in and out of the patients' houses. Every household along Grande Rue had at least one *malade*. Trucks pulled in beside the grocery stores, where room permitted, and unloaded dozens of cartons of *biscottes* manufactured in distant cities. The bakeries were shuttered and locked—all of them.

By midmorning on Monday the men from the Fourteenth Mobile Brigade of Montpellier, the *gendarmerie*, and the *inspecteurs des services de repression des fraudes* had swept into the village, along with the *chef de cabinet du préfet du Gard*, the chief administration office of the *département*. They were seen everywhere in the streets, collecting samples of the bread from each household, lifting two hundred grams of flour from each of the *boulangeries*, and placing the shops themselves under official seal.

For the first time, datelined Tuesday, August 21, 1951, the newspaper *La Marseillaise* published a small news item on page 6. It was the last page of the journal. The headline: LE PAIN DE PONT-SAINT-ESPRIT PROVOQUE DES INTOXICATIONS. UN MORT. In France, *intoxications* signified poisoning, not drunkenness. Ironically, on the front page a banner headline covered the main story throughout France of the day: The price of bread and bread products was increased by 23 percent.

There was very little detail given in the item about Pont-Saint-Esprit. "*Une grave affair d'intoxication alimentaire à Pont-Saint-Esprit a provoqué des multiples indispositions, non seulement dans cette commune du Gard, mais encore dans les villages voisins, tout au long de la vallée du Rhône,*" it began.

It went on to say that up through Monday, August 20, nearly 150 cases were being treated by the doctors, (the doctors had at that time actually counted nearly three hundred) and that M. Mison, age 62, had died in the hospital at Nîmes. It announced that an inquiry had been opened by the Parquet, the public prosecutor of Nîmes, as well as a judiciary investigation, to establish if all the victims had obtained their bread from the bakery of M. Briand, who was also himself ill, along with his wife and his helper. The item concluded:

"Actually, the evolution of the disease appears favorable, and it is no longer believed that any further deaths will follow."

The brunt of the investigation fell on the *cabinet* of the *juge d'instruction*—the examining magistrate—of the Court of Appeals of Nîmes, M. Perrier. No one could face a more massive or complex inquiry. To be coordinated were the public prosecutor, *le procureur de la République*, and his deputy, the Fourteenth Mobile Brigade, the *gendarmerie*, the local police, the local physicians, the *ministre de l'interieur, direction générale de la sûreté national*, the medical specialists and toxicologists to be called in, the Laboratoire Interrégional de Police Scientifique de Marseilles, the local authorities, the officials of the Union Meunière, the ministry of health of both the *département* of Gard and the Republic, the S.N.C.F. which had transported the flour in its freight cars; the directors and staffs of the hospitals, some three hundred witnesses and principals, and whatever other elements that might be uncovered. The most urgent priority at the moment was the lifting of the samples of bread and flour from the bakeries and the distribution center at Bagnols-Sur-Cèze, and the shipping of the cadavers of the animals from the farms surrounding Pont-Saint-Esprit, which had died after eating the bread, to the Laboratoire Interrégional de Police Scientifique. The logistics were not simple. Police swarmed through the town, interrogating the villagers and asking them to dig through garbage pails and trash baskets to find any bread, suspected or not. Each sample was to be carefully labeled and numbered. The corpses of the dogs, cats, and ducks were dumped into sacks to be rushed to Marseilles. Some had to be dug up from shallow graves.

An autopsy was immediately ordered on the body of M. Mison. Medical clues were desperately needed; his death might serve as a sacrifice for the living. The first step was for the protection of the health of the people. The second was to find out what negligence, fraud, or even criminal action was involved in a plague that was growing more mysterious by the hour.

Like everyone else involved in the mystery, the examining magistrate was fighting the same phantom enemy that had eluded the doctors, the patients, and the baker himself. Theories and rumors were everywhere. Those that occurred to the authorities had for the most part already been advanced by the townspeople, whose shrewd native instincts were as sharp as those of the experts. Whenever a theory was discussed at the meetings, at the police conferences, in the medical offices, the news leaked out, and the rumors took on a new fire, a new sense of urgency, as if the mystery were now solved, and the definitive answer had been found and backed up by authority.

And so it was that by the time Monday evening came, the atmosphere among the villagers was charged with certainty: *It was arsenic*. The sacks of flour, said the word passed from person to person, had been drenched with liquid arsenic en route to the village. Where it came from and what kind of arsenic it was did not matter. The truth, the absolute truth, was that it was arsenic. Everybody who had even nibbled the bread would die sooner or later, within weeks, and there was nothing that medicine could do about it. The rumor spread so quickly, so forcefully, that people went home, gathered their families together, and knelt in prayer. Many sobbed and cried as they came off the streets to bring the news to their families. Hardly anyone knew or would accept the fact that the source of the rumor was an offhand remark by a *gendarme*, thinking out loud to himself as he collected a sample of bread from a villager. His speculation had been transformed into a pronouncement of unimpeachable authority, yet there was no foundation whatever to it.

This theory had already been seriously considered by the doctors at first and by the police and toxicologists later. Arsenic compounds were used everywhere in the vineyards and farms for the treatment of vines and as insecticides. Some of the symptoms of arsenic poisoning had, in fact, been present: low blood pressure, depressed respiration, convulsions. But other symptoms were definitely not present, such as garlic odor of the breath, projectile vomiting with the presence of blood, rapid weak pulse, and others. More importantly, arsenic poisoning is easily traced.

During the first days of the sickness the signs were so variable that there could be as many theories as there were symptoms. By the time the police arrived in the village, the fifth day after the illness had first appeared, the dominant symptom was insomnia. This was almost universal among the victims, along with a marked dehydration.

As the symptoms developed, the doctors slowly realized that the ergot theory—the poisoning from a mold forming on certain grains—was becoming a more logical and distinct possibility, in spite of the fact that historical ergotism was thought to be a thing of the past, a relic of the Middle Ages which had had a few fitful outbursts in the eighteenth century and the beginning of the nineteenth but rarely in the twentieth. The terror it had provoked in the Middle Ages was of such magnitude that the plague was called *mal des ardents,* meaning "sickness of the burning and the scorched," and *le feu de St. Antoine,* "St. Anthony's Fire," because only supplications to St. Anthony were supposed to have had any effect when the tragedy struck. Entire villages had been stricken then with the most horrifying and terrifying madness, and the scenes in the village streets were of unbelievable chaos as hundreds became psychotic almost at a single moment.

Psychic disturbance, a definitive symptom of ergotism, was certainly in evidence now, but the doctors knew that these current disturbances might be ordinary delirium, and besides, they had not shown any indication of appearing in the form of the characteristic major outbreak. Furthermore, the physicians were not at all anxious to announce the possibility of such a rare and mysterious disease; there was no effective method of treatment for it, and they did not want to alarm the population. All that was really known about historical ergotism was that it resulted from an unknown poison of the ergot alkaloid series.

One doctor, speculating about the possibility of historical ergotism, mumbled in ironic humor that it would be extremely difficult to treat the disease, if *ergotisme historique* were indeed the cause, because the only medical research papers were illuminated manuscripts of the fifteenth century. He was exaggerating only slightly. There *was* a more modern and lengthy treatise on the plague, written as late as 1887, in the *Dictionnaire Encyclopédie de Science Médecine,* which described in vivid terms the utter savagery and paroxysms experienced by a village struck by ergotism that resulted from mold on the grain from which bread had been made. The picture painted was not a comforting one.

Judge Perrier's first ordinance was a set of instructions to M. Henri Ollivier, professor of the School of Medicine of the University of Marseilles, and director of the police scientific laboratory there, to determine the cause of the mass illness through exhaustive toxicological tests on the bread, flour, sacks, and viscera specimens supplied by the doctors and the *gendarmes*.

Professor Ollivier was faced with an overwhelming job. In its simplest form toxicology is slow, laborious, and exacting; in the present case it was to involve up to three hundred samples of bread, scores of flour samples, the bodies of dozens of domestic animals, and tragically, human viscera. The sheer job of organizing and cataloguing the material was arduous and time-consuming. The number of tests, both toxicologically classical and specific, called for more time than was available if the doctors were to be supplied urgent guidelines with which to work. In addition, each test consumed a considerable portion of an individual sample, so that often there was not enough bulk to the sample to permit all the classical and specific tests necessary to arrive at a definitive conclusion.

It was not only necessary to analyze the samples chemically; portions of the samples would also have to be injected or fed to laboratory test animals to observe the toxicity on a living organism. There were no short cuts. Also, some poisons are unstable and short-lived. Their potency disintegrates rapidly, leaving little or no traces. Bread, especially, dries up very quickly, and with it, the important evidence.

The pressures on the laboratory team working with Professor Ollivier were nerve-wracking. Further tragedy in the village was hanging in the balance; the doctors were working without intelligent information. Time was paramount, but a mistaken or hasty analysis was worse. From the start the team was unwittingly caught in a vise, and like the others, was fighting against the same phantom of obscurity that had marked the tragedy from the beginning.

M. Ollivier took a great deal of pride in his work. Some even felt the pride was excessive. Dark, lean, and intense, the young doctor began the work with the uncomfortable knowledge that the lives of an entire town were dependent on him and what he was able to discover.

At the same time the Office National Interprofessionnel des Céréales, better known as the O.N.I.C., ordered some samples to be sent to the Laboratoire Régional des Subsistances Militaires in Marseilles, to conduct an independent investigation and to help expedite the process of trying to discover the elusive cause. In contrast to the Union Meunière, the O.N.I.C. was a governmental agency, which regulated the work of the private corporation. The contract between the private monopoly (the Union Meunière) and the government agency (the O.N.I.C.) was complex; even lawyers shuddered at its legal labyrinths. Both, however, were deeply involved in the outcome of the toxicological tests, and both were to be drawn deeper and deeper into the case as it progressed.

When the men from the Fourteenth Mobile Brigade—including Commissioner Georges Sigaud, chief of the unit, and Inspector Étienne Vacher—arrived at M. Briand's shop, M. Briand was in a state of emotional shock. For over thirty years he had prized his reputation for making good bread. In a single baking, that reputation seemed to dissolve. The flour, *la farine*, as they called it, had changed without warning from doubtful to deadly. The questioning by the police was polite but harsh. The charges of involuntary homicide were already officially issued against "X," and there was no time for more than the barest of civilities.

Under their questioning, M. Briand re-created the entire scene of the night and morning of August 15–16: the borrowing of the bread from the other bakers, the preparation and baking of the three *fournées*, the mixing of the various flours, the color and texture of the batter. What other products beside the flour were used? Was anything different used that night of August 15 than on other nights? Were there any insecticides around the shop? Where were the water pipes?

There would be more questioning to follow. At the moment the main interest was the shop itself, and the investigators examined every inch of it. Samples of the water, yeast, and salt were labeled and seized. There were no insecticides or fungicides. M. Briand had never used any other chemicals or materials to fortify his bread, and nothing at all suspect was found in the search.

The investigation fanned out quickly to Bagnols-sur-Cèze, and to M. Bousquet. Only on Monday, August 20, had the samples of the originally suspected flour been sent to the Union Meunière. M. Bousquet had become tired of waiting for their instructions or for a representative to come and collect the samples, as they were required to do by contract. The previous cases of mild illness resulting from the bread sold by M. Monier, M. Griotti, and M. Jaussent now came prominently to the surface as the investigation broadened. The Seventeenth Brigade Régionale de Police Judicaire in Limoges went into action in the north to begin the inquiry there.

On Tuesday morning, August 21, another meeting was held at the Hôtel de Ville in the office of Mayor Hebrard. The three local doctors, not having been to bed for over a hundred hours, were literally on the brink of total exhaustion. Strangely, both Dr. Vieu and Dr. Channac, who had eaten the suspected bread, were able to withstand the strain better than Dr. Gabbai. Their illness had now reached the stage of many of their own patients: almost total insomnia supported by an accompanying unnatural force and energy. An official pronouncement was made for the first time: A collective poisoning, affecting many of the townspeople, has been determined; M. Mison of Carsan has died; others are seriously ill; all the best medical facilities are being put to use to combat the illness. The fears of the villagers were somewhat placated by another rumor that was circulating now along Grande Rue: M. Mison had died from a "collapse of the heart and blood vessels," and only the very elderly, who were soon to die anyway, were in any danger. The fact that severe cardiovascular reactions had been noted in victims of all ages was not yet generally known.

By evening Professor Gaston Giraud of the School of Medicine of the University of Montpellier had arrived, along with Professor Recordier of the University of Marseilles. A second meeting was held, including the examining magistrate and the assistant to the prefect of the *département*. It was immediately decided to bring in several interns from the hospital at Nîmes to assist the sagging and exhausted local doctors. Professors Giraud and Recordier would analyze all the data so far collected, as well as examine a large number of patients to attempt a clear diagnosis.

The meetings, the analyses of the data, and the laboratory tests were necessary, but they did nothing to correct the situation at the immediate moment. Back at the Moulin farmhouse Mme. Moulin was struggling against the now standard feeling of alternating total wakefulness and total exhaustion. She had not closed her eyes for four days. At lunch time on Tuesday, when her husband and son came in from the vineyards, each was in continued pain and distress. It was obvious that neither husband nor son would go back to work in the vineyards; every worker in the Moulin vineyards, in fact, was sick, and only four of the total of nine were able to be on their feet.

"All my joints pain me," said her husband. "My ankles. My knees. Everything. I must go to bed."

Young Joseph was almost doubled up in pain. "I can't go on like this," he said. "I can't stand it."

Alarmed, Mme. Moulin helped each of them into his bed, brought them *infusion de thyme*, and found that she herself was shivering so fiercely that she had to wrap herself in a blanket even though the midday August sun was broiling. After a few moments even the blanket was insufficient. She piled the fireplace high with faggots, lighted them, and huddled close by as the sweat poured from her. Her cold and shivering increased. She piled more fuel on the fire until it frightened her with its crackling intensity. But it did no good whatever.

The first of the major convulsions came that evening. Both M. Moulin and young Joseph were writhing on their beds, forearms snapping toward their shoulders, knees jerking upward without cease. Mme. Moulin, now so weak herself that she could hardly get out of her chair by the fireplace, struggled to their bedsides, helpless in her attempt to keep them covered or give them succor. A neighbor who had dropped by several hours before had promised to get the doctor, but he had not yet arrived.

How many hours—it seemed days—Mme. Moulin had to wait, she did not know. When the doctor did arrive, he found Mme. Moulin crying almost hysterically beside her husband's bed; both husband and son were wracked with convulsions. He ordered an ambulance through a neighbor, who had to drive two kilometers to the nearest phone, administered intravenous sedatives to all three, and waited, despairingly, to see if there would be any effect. There was none.

When Mme. Moulin had recovered some of her composure, the doctor told her, "All of you must go to the hospital. You are too far away here to be taken care of. You must."

"But *Docteur*," said Mme. Moulin, "there is the vineyard. There is no one to take care of the farm. We cannot all go."

The doctor thought a moment, then said, "There is no other choice."

Mme. Moulin, still shaking from cold and heat at the same

time, pleaded with him. "My daughter will arrive here soon. She will take care of the place. Please, can't I wait here until she comes? It will be tomorrow."

The doctor assented, but insisted that both husband and son be taken immediately. It took two hours for the ambulance from the Clinique Cloy, at Villeneuve-les-Avignon, to arrive. The last words Mme. Moulin heard as her son was lifted into the ambulance along with her husband were, "Mother, I think I am dying. My heart is going to stop."

Any words from her husband were drowned out by the shrieking of the ambulance as it burst out of the farmyard on the way to the hospital.

Alone, Mme. Moulin sat by the kitchen table, her heart wrung with sorrow, her body wracked with pain. Again, time went by uncounted, but she did not close her eyes, she did not sleep, and there were no more tears to cry.

She was aware, quite suddenly, of the kitchen door opening, then closing. There was a doctor standing in the doorway, but it was not her doctor, nor was he one she had ever seen before. He was dressed in a black suit and wore black shoes and a white shirt with a black tie. He carried a black bag in his hand. He was silent, not speaking and not moving. Her eyes traveled slowly up from his shoes to his shoulders, and at last to his head.

There was no face there, only a skull—a *tête de mort*. The empty eye sockets stared at her blankly. She screamed. The figure of the unknown doctor did not move. She reached for an iron pot lying in front of her on the kitchen table. She hurled it at the *tête de mort* with all the force she could gather. It passed through the head and shoulders of the motionless doctor and splintered a wooden panel of the door. The pot clattered to the floor at the feet of the doctor, but the feet were no longer there. Nor was the rest of the doctor, nor the skull. She screamed again, but there was no one around to hear her. She knew that she was hallucinating, but the hallucination was so vivid it might just as well be reality.

It grew slowly, what Mayor Hebrard was to call "the nightmare that has come to our village!" There were signs of it gathering each day and each hour until it arrived. Not even the doctors, inured as they were to the unexpected crises that broke out on every side of them, were prepared for what was going to happen.

The villagers certainly were not, in spite of the apprehension, the panic, the sorrow, and the hopelessness. The signs that gathered pointed unerringly in the same direction, but they gave no indication of the magnitude the nightmare was to assume.

There had been Mme. Moulin and her doctor with the "head of death." There had been the tigers and the blood dripping from the ceiling that little Marie-Joseph Carle had seen. There had been the strange compulsion of her father, as he found himself craving for bead curtains for the flies to rest on, and counting the six window panes in his bedroom endlessly now, for over a day and a night. There had been the young engineer with a compulsion to walk, and to think of potatoes. There had been the strange, indescribable colors seen by M. Delacquis, and the expanding and contracting horizons as he cycled home from his office to La Villette that day that now seemed centuries ago. There was also his compulsion to write, day and night, without cease now.

Not all of these indications were known in total, even to the doctors. Not all the cases of dogs, cats, and ducks had been reported, but in sixteen villages in and around Pont-Saint-Esprit, the ducks had also strutted like penguins; the cats had screeched, clawed, and drawn their motionless hindquarters along the floor; the dogs had crushed their teeth on rocks, or made senseless attacks on trees until their teeth fell out with the bark they ripped from them. Not all of the animals had died, but many had. These all were separated items, however, not joined in any one tapestry which could be quickly and easily discerned.

In hindsight, the panoramic view of all the happenings could be observed in perspective. It is then easy to say: It was all so obvious. Why did it require such a long time to realize the full impact of what was growing? But working under pressure, as the doctors and authorities were, the building blocks of the tragic structure, slowly forming in front of their eyes, were in fragments. An investigator examined only one brick at a time. The architect's plans and drawings were nowhere in sight. And the bricks, or other individual construction units, were in scattered piles; some hidden, some unrecognizable, some uncounted. And further, there was the element of incredibility. What was shaping up was so hard to conceive that there was a natural tendency to reject the evidence at hand. It was so unbelievable, the psyche could not accept it.

M. and Mme. Marcel Boudenne, for instance, had no idea what

was happening at the beginning. Together, they were proprietors of their combined hat-and-sporting-goods store, enjoying the leisurely chats with their clients, planning some day to move the shop to the wide vistas of the Boulevard Gambetta, away from the crowded quarters just off the Grande Rue by the place de l'Hotel de Ville. M. Boudenne, a warm and affable townsman, was also the local correspondent for several newspapers. Knowledgeable and more worldly than the average *Spiritpontain,* he watched the symptoms grow with awe and uncertainty, but also with a journalistic sense of detachment. He agreed with the doctors, as the situation became more serious, that extensive reportage would only contribute to more hysteria and panic, and held back his releases until it was no longer possible. Neither he nor his plump, congenial wife could understand the time when she was overwhelmed with a compulsion to punch him as hard as she could, yet without feeling any anger whatever. One night she woke him up to tell him just that, and together they laughed about it. At length, when the compulsion persisted, he suggested that she let go with a series of friendly punches, which she did, feeling better afterward. It became their own private joke; nothing more serious was made of it, and the strange and amusing compulsion soon stopped. There were many incidents like this, happening throughout the village, but neither the doctors nor the authorities were aware of them. They simply remained family jokes in the privacy of the home and were, it turned out, the extremely mild aberrations of those who were lucky enough not to be among the more seriously stricken of the village.

Nearly all the people who were to become principals in the drama were reasonably stable and normal folk. Their lives had been no more disturbed than those of any collection of people living in a village and working, loving, and living together, along with the common stresses and problems that all life carries with it.

Joseph Moulin and his son were held in the greatest esteem in the area. M. Delacquis was loved by all who knew him. M. Testevin was a tower of strength and reliability. Emile's charm and strength was legendary. M. Carle was a model example of the successful proprietor who provided for both his family and the welfare needs of the community. M. Sauvet's sparkling eyes and personality were known throughout the village with affection. M. Mison was particularly mourned because of the love and respect in which he had been held. Charles Pommier, living in the little village of Lamotte, just across the ancient bridge, on the other side of the Rhône, ranked with all these in his standing in the community, and was a close friend of Mayor Hebrard.

This is why, when he symbolically became the first authentic harbinger of what was to follow, the shock was so great. A sixty-six-year-old widower, he had been among the first to be stricken, and hard. He lay on his bed for many days, wakeful but too weak to move. His prostration and insomnia were total, and he was cared for lovingly, but despairingly, by his son and neighbors.

On Wednesday, nearly a week after the first cases had been recorded, he lay on his bed, still prostrate, weak, and uncommunicative. It happened suddenly, so suddenly that his son, outside the house in the garden, was momentarily paralyzed with confusion.

M. Pommier shot forth from his bed, roaring and screaming. Disheveled and demented, he screamed out the window that his enemies were coming to get him. There was foam on his mouth; his eyes were wild and unfocused. He disappeared from the window, as his son ran toward the house. Reaching the front door, the son pushed it, but it did not budge. He pounded on it and begged his father to let him in, but the only answer was more demented shouts and screams. He ran to the back door, but it too was now locked. Inside, his father—shouting that he was being attacked by some unseen, unknown enemy—was piling furniture up against the doors and windows.

When the *gendarmes* arrived, he was at his bedroom window, shotgun in hand, brandishing it at the approaching enemy that only he alone could see. The police deployed around the house, keeping out of sight, out of range of the gun. At the window, still foaming and roaring, M. Pommier screamed at the police to come out from behind their barriers and help fight his enemies. The police called to him, telling him to put down his gun; that they would help him if he would do that. Slowly, doubtfully, he lowered the gun, now becoming calmer. With caution, the police drew toward the house, then in a sudden surge moved to the door and broke it in.

Chests, chairs, and tables were piled against it. The inside of the house was a shambles. Carefully, the police made their way up the stairs, keeping low and against the wall. The bedroom door was also barricaded. M. Pommier was still screaming that his enemies were after him; that if the police were not careful, they would also be killed.

Again, the inside door was smashed in, the furniture barricade pushed back. M. Pommier was huddled in the corner, away from the window, sobbing quietly. The shotgun lay across his knees. Cautiously, the police approached him. Then, with a sudden movement he seized a candle, laughing wildly, and began a strange and macabre dance, with awkward, jerky contortions. The police watched, in cautious silence. Then he stopped, stared at them, and sunk down on a chair. Quiet now, he willingly handed them the gun, saying nothing. They straightened the furniture, tenderly put him back in the bed. He did not resist. Then, with wild, loud laughter, shrieking and high-pitched, he screamed:

"Tomorrow, tomorrow I am getting married! Do you hear? Do you understand? Tomorrow, I marry! If you wish, you must all come to the wedding!"

This was the prelude, the harbinger.

The second was an eleven-year-old boy. Suddenly, everyone became his enemy. His mother, approaching him to try to calm him down, was abruptly faced with a raging child who hurled himself on her, scratching and pummelling her face and arms. Her husband, helpless and prostrate on his bed, was in the middle of a convulsive fit of hallucinations at the same time. She freed herself, ran for help from her neighbors. Father and son were rushed to l'Hôtel-Dieu in the same ambulance.

The third flash of heat lightning, before the storm struck, was M. Sauvet, the popular *garagiste,* in his forties, married, and now sick for several days. His wife, administering endless *infusions* of dried lime flowers, prayed that some kind of improvement would rouse him from his condition of total lethargy and listlessness. The intolerable burning in his stomach and esophagus had diminished somewhat, but the weakness and the lack of sleep were continuing. It was about nine in the evening when she saw him sit up suddenly in the bed, breathing heavily, muscles and arms flexing, his eyes with their widened pupils staring directly ahead, totally unaware of his surroundings. Then, with an abrupt motion, he seized the square pillow case and slowly ripped it down the middle. Quickly, he turned to the sheets, the blankets. He firmly pushed her away as she tried to stop him. Taking the sheet first, he ripped it into shred after shred, then the blankets, then he attacked the bedstead itself, pounding it into splinters. All the while, his visage was smiling, pleasantly and confidently, as if this were a delightful and gratifying pastime. Totally unable to stop him, Mme. Sauvet crouched behind the shattered bedstead in hopeless desperation.

M. Sauvet was not aware of that. Because clearly in his own perception he was not in his bedroom anymore. He was in the circus, performing the act of a strong man in front of an admiring throng. He was bending iron bars double, as the applause in his ears grew louder and louder. He was ripping sheets of thick steel down the middle, as if they were made of cardboard. He was taking huge timbers and breaking them over his knees. At every stage of the act, the audience, right in front of his eyes, was growing more appreciative. He bowed in modest acknowledgement again and again. As he accepted the roaring applause and prepared to return to his dressing room, he slowly became aware that the audience was nonexistent, that it consisted only of his wife, huddled in the corner of the bedroom, in tears. The bent iron bar was nothing more than a ripped pillow case; the steel plates were the shreds that were left of the sheets; the giant timbers, the splintered remnants of the bedstead. As his awareness returned, he became conscious that all of this had been a wild delusion, and he was filled with remorse. Yet what he envisaged had been so real it might as well have happened. His anxiety arose when he could not explain it to his frightened wife. He fell back weakly on the twisted ribbons of the sheets, wondering what was going to happen next, pleading with his wife to forgive him for an impulse and an event that was as inexplicable to him as it was to her.

The *crise* of M. Sauvet overlapped another outbreak by the little daughter of M. Carle. Again the tigers returned, this time more menacing than ever. While her father lay on his bed, hopelessly and endlessly counting the window panes, he was so gripped by his *idée fixe* that he could not hear her shrieks and moans. Mme. Carle, halfway between the two bedrooms, could hear both the booming monotonous counting of her husband and the screaming of her daughter. She ran to the child's bedroom to find her thrashing her arms and legs wildly, yelling that the tiger was now at her throat and going to rip her to pieces. So violent was her lashing out that she continually struck her head and her arms on the bedstead and wall, bruising herself badly in the process.

The doctor, notified by a neighbor, had already called for the local ambulance before he arrived, phoning the hospital at Avignon to expect the young girl's arrival. What was most immediate was to save the child from seriously injuring herself in her hallucinations. With the help of Mme. Carle, he cut strips of sheeting, and it took the strength of the two of them to lash the child to the bed. There she lay crying out that the blood dropping from the ceiling was drowning her as the tigers were biting off her feet.

It began at La Villette with M. Delacquis. For days now, he had lain silent and sleepless on his bed. Mme. Testevin was preparing for another sleepless night herself, as she had for the past week. Things had settled down now into a grotesque routine. In the mornings, with the help of the Rigaud sisters, she would strip the beds of all four of the *malades*, the sheets drenched with sweat and the odor of mice, which still persisted. While the sisters made up the new beds, she would boil the sheets in a huge vat, soak them in *eau de javel*, take them out to the stone well, pound them and drench them in the clear spring water until they were fresh and clean, then hang them up to dry. Then she would greet a parade of neighbors bringing gifts and food to her to help her in her trouble. But the food was useless: No one in any of the four rooms wanted any whatever. They were able to take, at uncertain times, Mme. Testevin's favorite *infusion de verveine*, an herb tea of her own concoction, or some hot beef bouillon. But each *malade* had to be spoon fed like a baby, unable to help and more frequently resisting the succor she tried to bring them.

She had already taken all the winter blankets out of their storage bags, making endless rounds to cover and uncover the sick, as they alternately shivered and sweated in excruciating extremes. Because of the emergency pressures on the village physicians it fell on her and the Rigaud sisters to administer injections of vitamins for holding back the serious consequences of the *malades*' lack of nutrition, and shots of gardenal in a futile attempt to bring calmness and sleep which had not yet arrived for any of the four stricken persons.

By afternoon the Rigaud sisters had left, Mme. Testevin remained alone to try to attend and comfort the others. By nightfall she would begin her rounds of the patients, moving from one bedroom to the other, and trying to sleep in chairs in the rooms for brief moments, spending about fifteen minutes in each room in an endless cycle. But she, too, had been stricken, and she found she could not sleep, even though she desperately needed to. The sleeplessness had become actually painful now, a burning pain that made the eyes sting and ache with every blink of the lids.

This night began as any of the last several nights. She stopped first at the bedroom of M. Delacquis, at the top of the stairs. As usual, he was propped up in bed, tablet on his knees, writing. Usually well-groomed, he was now disheveled. He did not seem to be aware of her entering. She brought with her a tray with another classic remedy, a cup of *tisane d'orge*, or barley-water.

Softly she said to him: "You must try to sleep, M. Delacquis. But before you do, take some of this."

His eyes seemed to come back into focus for a moment, and he said, "Have you been able to find me the newspaper?"

Every day he asked for the newspaper. And every day Mme. Testevin tried to mumble some excuse, because the story of the sickness was just now beginning to dominate the headlines. Only that day they were screaming about the emotion in the village growing hour by hour, that all along the Grande Rue there was panic since the death of M. Mison, that medicines were useless, that even the strongest were being stricken, as young Joseph Moulin and his father had been rushed to the hospital at Villeneuve-lès-Avignon.

"Perhaps tomorrow," she told M. Delacquis. "I have not been able to go down to the village for many days."

"I would be so grateful," M. Delacquis replied, and he went back to his writing pad. It was filled with tiny, precise script, and each day Mme. Testevin had someone bring him a new pad from the village. Without his pad, he became very disturbed. With it, he seemed to achieve some kind of therapeutic sublimation that brought him reasonable calm. She never asked him what he was writing, so delicate was the balance of his emotional state. But she could see that it was for the most part in carefully written verse, in spite of the apparent disarray of his mind.

She smoothed his pillows, wiped his forehead and lips with a cool, damp washcloth, left the room, and returned in a moment with a small vase of freshly cut flowers. She kept flowers in every room, and she now arranged these neatly and placed them on a small table below the crucifix on the wall. M. Delacquis had slid back into himself again, writing with the same obsessional intensity he had been demonstrating all day and all night for the past several days.

At the doorway she stopped, looked at his strained, thin face, and came back toward his bed again. "You could not *try* to go to sleep?" she asked, knowing from her own sleeplessness how futile the question was. "What if I turned the light out for you?"

Lost completely in his thoughts, M. Delacquis did not reply. His pencil seemed to be moving almost automatically along the paper. Mme. Testevin, looking down at his fingers, saw that they were red and sore from the pressure of the pencil. "Your fingers," she said. "They are so sore. Perhaps . . ."

He was paying no attention to her and continued to write. She gave up her effort and went out the door and down the tile-floored hallway to the room of Mme. Dezeuzes.

There was a small light on beside the bed. Mme. Dezeuzes, sweat pouring from her face, was lying on her side. She was staring at the wall and sobbing. She had been sobbing day and night, also without sleep, for nearly a week. She would not talk or communicate. The sobs were low and soft, always, but particularly tragic to Mme. Testevin because they were so pathetic. She placed fresh flowers beside the bed, again wiped the face of Mme. Dezeuzes, automatically straightened the bed clothes, and went on into the Testevin bedroom.

M. Testevin was lying in his bed, on his back, wide open eyes, staring at the ceiling. He had hardly moved from this position over the past week. "He lies like a dead man," Mme. Testevin would mumble to herself.

He would not respond to anything. She smoothed his hair, washed his face gently, kissed him tenderly on the forehead. He did not move, did not appear to see her, even though his eyes were wide open. This was most painful to Mme. Testevin, because it seemed like death itself, with the eyes staring upward, the hands motionless on his chest, the total muteness.

"*Mon cher, mon cher, mon cher,*" she mumbled, then went down to the dining room to Emile, now rolling back and forth on his cot, moaning as he always did, day and night, all through the week.

Emile seemed always in pain, and was completely out of touch with his surroundings. To give him tea or water was the most difficult of tasks, because it would invariably spill on the sheets, already wet with the constant sweat that all four of the patients exuded day and night. Emile was the only one who resisted almost any aid brought to him. It became a struggle between the will of Mme. Testevin with the wash cloth or a cup of tea, and that of Emile, who attempted to avoid them. This night, Mme. Testevin noted, was a little easier. He sipped his tea, permitted her to wipe down his face, and dry his sweat. But when she was finished, he went back to his moaning and tossing without cease.

Alone in the kitchen, Mme. Testevin brewed herself a cup of tea, and prayed for her four *malades* in the house. With the door closed, she could find at least a small semblance of silence, although from the other rooms of the house came the same sounds that she had been hearing all during the week, a strange orchestration from four different directions. From the rooms of M. Delacquis and her husband, she would hear only occasional muffled sighs at rare moments. From Mme. Dezeuzes' room she would hear the steady, relentless sobbing, which never stopped. From Emile, on the cot in the dining room, she would hear the constant moaning, mostly soft, but frequently loud and intense, blasting the night silence in the large, darkened house. And when Emile's moans would increase, so would the sobbing of Mme. Dezeuzes. This was a rhythmic and almost predictable pattern, a pattern she was now accepting as part of a macabre routine which had no end in sight.

It was because of her acceptance of this routine that the first signal of something different developing startled her so much. From the room of M. Delacquis came a sharp, piercing, hideous screech. It was shattering beyond her memory of such a sound. She rushed up the stairs to his room. He was sitting on the edge of the bed, pointing wildly to the window.

"*Regardez!*" he shouted. "*Regardez la boule de feu! Il se rapproche! Il nous tue!*"

Still screaming, he crumbled to the floor, slid half under the bed, cowering, hiding his head under his arms. Mme. Testevin rushed to him, tried to pull him out from under, but he thrashed at her wildly, wedging himself further under, screaming that a huge ball of fire was coming toward them, was going to kill them. Mme. Testevin tugged at his arm, without success. She felt overwhelmed with helplessness, retreated to the center of the room and begged God for strength and guidance.

It was then that she heard the crash in the dining room below her. It was followed by a moment of silence, then another harrowing scream, this time from Emile. Then shouts and a series of thuds which seemed to shake the house. Quickly, she grabbed a blanket from the bed, squeezed it between the bottom of the springs and the cowering M. Delacquis, and ran downstairs.

The dining room was a shambles. The table upset, the chest pushed in the center of the floor. Emile was roaring, clawing at the air, backing into the corner. The beasts, the lions, the claws, he was shouting, were coming at him from every side. Their heads were enormous, their eyes staring at him, ready to kill him. He was throwing dishes at them, breaking chairs against the wall, attempting to kill them, fighting a phantom fight for his life. Summoning all her courage, for Emile was among the strongest of men, she went toward him, grabbed his flailing arms, and tried to push him back to the bed. He threw off her grasp, screaming a warning that she too would be killed by the beasts surrounding them. She fought back, grabbed him again. Again he pushed her back against the overturned table. Upstairs, she could hear Mme. Dezeuzes suddenly breaking into louder hysterical cries, accompanied by the horrifying shrieks of M. Delacquis.

Emile continued raging around the room, thrashing his arms in every direction, overturning his bed and beating off imaginary animals. Mme. Testevin, overwhelmed, dropped her head on the edge of the overturned table and sobbed.

As M. Pommier barricaded himself within his house to fight off his enemies with his shotgun, as the eleven-year-old boy attacked his mother, as M. Sauvet ripped his bed clothing to shreds, as

Mme. Testevin faced her unbelievable nightmare at La Villette, as the little Marie-Joseph Carle was screaming in the ambulance on her way to the hospital at Avignon, the villagers were not aware of these scattered events. The police and the doctors knew, and the signs were ominous. But to the villagers as a whole, the sickness was simply continuing its uncomfortable course without change. There was the terrible fear among the populace, and it was mounting in the face of the mystery surrounding the disease. But the strange phenomenon of the *euphorie béate* continued to rise in crescendo. It was not until nearly midnight on Friday, August 24, 1951, that the terrifying and fast-multiplying proportions and ramifications of the plague became clearly evident to the entire village, in spite of all the doctors and authorities could do to keep the news of what was happening—and worse, what was about to happen—from creating a panic so great that the efforts to fight the enemy would be lost in total hysteria and confusion.

About one hour before midnight, Friday, August 24, 1951, *l'-éclosion brutale*—the savage breaking-out—began. It came at the peak of the tide of the *euphorie béate,* and in shocking contrast to it. All during the week the scattered events had foreshadowed it. In spite of this, the doctors and the authorities, had no available means to control it or to soften its blow.

SIX

THE NIGHTMARE began spilling out *en masse* in both the village itself and the towns and farms surrounding Pont-Saint-Esprit, as far as ten kilometers away, as if some cosmic signal had been given to unleash a diabolic tidal wave. Some say it was far worse in the narrow streets of the village, where the shrieks and screams were heard echoing and resounding against the walls of the houses, ripping through the night air at unpredictable intervals. Mixed with the cries of anguish was the ominous *wee-waw-wee-waw-wee-waa* of the French ambulance sirens, the screech of their tires. Others say that it was worse on the isolated farms, where wives alone faced husbands and brothers in uncontrollable tantrums, with no help at hand; or where husbands were forced to use brute strength to keep their wives or sisters or mothers from tearing themselves to pieces.

In this region, neighbor to the ghostly caves of Les Baux, which had inspired Dante to write his *Inferno,* the Hôtel-Dieu, the ancient hospital of Pont-Saint-Esprit, became a scene as vivid as any in Dante's story. There was no mass hysteria inspiring the victims themselves. The widely separated *malades* were no more conscious of what was happening to the others in distant villages then if they had been in another country. The victims in the crowded streets were mentally removed from the surroundings before the outbreak could influence them. Afterward, they lived only in their own worlds.

There *was* mass hysteria, but it grew among the people who were *not* stricken, as they watched their loved ones and neighbors suddenly become violent and implacable strangers. But the two were clearly separated: Psychosis from physical disease; hysteria from sheer fright. The suffocating feeling of being trapped was insufferable. The overwhelming fear, "where and when will it strike next?" dominated everyone. In turn, came the feeling of distrust—of neighbors, of friends, of members of the family. A normal person one minute could be a demented maniac the next. They watched this happen in front of their eyes. Even those who had not eaten the bread were frozen with fear. There was no guarantee that the bread was the cause, only a speculation. Some walked through the streets clutching crucifixes and beads. The exodus from the village increased in volume, as cars and trucks made their way out of the streets to other towns, other houses in foreign cities.

One of the first outbreaks in full public view came late evening on Friday. Charles Veladaire, a worker on the Mondragon project, broke suddenly away from a group of his sleepless friends, who were talking in hushed tones that night, and he let out out a piercing scream. He ran from the place de l'Hôtel de Ville, down the rue Beauregard toward the Rhône, his startled friends chasing him, calling to him to come back. At the Quai de Luynes he stopped on the edge of the river and warned his friends to stand back.

"Don't touch me! Stand back! Stand back all of you," he yelled. "I am dead, do you hear? I am dead! My head is made of copper, and I have snakes in my stomach! They are burning, burning, burning!"

He turned to face the swirling current of the Rhône, which was dark, ominous, and turbulent beneath him. Two of his friends approached him cautiously.

"Stand back! Don't come near me!" he yelled again. "The snakes are burning me, don't you understand? They'll burn you to death!"

He turned again and prepared to jump. One friend, moving

swiftly, tackled him at the knees. The other, rushing to their side, pulled both of them back as they grappled on the edge of the stone embankment. All three were poised precariously until the rest of the group could reach them. The scuffle continued until it moved back on the darkened quay under the pressure of the mass of men. There were seven others, and even then they could barely hold Veladaire down. He broke away once and dashed madly toward the bank again, but he was trapped and held down until his struggling subsided. On his feet, they guided him along the rue Saint-Jacques and the Boulevard Carnot to the hospital. Twice he broke away again, and twice he was recaptured, bruised and bleeding.

Sister Négre, in the hospital Hôtel-Dieu doorway, watched them approach. Her heart was filled with despair. Already the hospital was jammed with desperately ill people. Three were already in a dangerously psychotic state. The hospital was not equipped to handle this type of case. She was a mass of bruises from trying to hold down the other cases. A fourth psychotic was too much for their facilities, but there were also the duty and responsibility which she never shirked. She held open the door as the group, still scuffling with their friend, moved into the echoing stone hallway, where his shrieks were amplified by the hollow somberness of the ancient building.

Dr. Gabbai later was to call this night "my night of the Apocalypse." He arrived at the hospital around eleven, after Sister Négre had phoned him about the arrival of Joseph Puche. M. Puche was a former aviator, a strong and intelligent man, who arrived gasping for breath and in obviously serious condition. He was placed in a bed on the second floor. The other floors had long since been filled up by the increase in serious victims who could not be cared for at their homes.

Parking his car outside the hospital on the Boulevard Carnot, behind the cars of Dr. Vieu and Dr. Channac, who were already there, Dr. Gabbai looked up at the windows. Every light in the building was blazing. Behind the windows the figures of the sisters moving back and forth across the wards could be seen. There was no night and day now in the hospital. The patients could not sleep because of the mass insomnia, and the sisters could not sleep because of the demands of their wakeful patients.

Suddenly a form appeared in a second-floor window. It was a

man, and he was gesticulating wildly. In a moment he was on the sill. Two sisters were behind him now, begging him to get back in the room. Each time they reached out, he slashed their hands away. It was Joseph Puche, the ex-aviator.

"Watch!" he shouted to the dark streets below. "Look at me! I'm an airplane, do you understand? I'm an airplane, and I can fly!"

Dr. Gabbai was transfixed in horror. The two sisters were begging the man in the name of God to come back in the building.

"I can fly! Don't all of you *believe* me?" he yelled. "Watch me!"

All of this had taken less than ten seconds. With no further warning, he jumped, arms outstretched as if they were the wings of an airplane.

He soared through the air, landed on the Boulevard Carnot, almost telescoping both his legs. He screamed in agony. Dr. Gabbai ran to his side. The sisters ran out of the hospital. As the doctor reached his side, the blood was already soaking through his hospital gown from the greenstick fractures. Then, incredibly, he rose up on his shattered legs and ran full speed down the boulevard. Several stunned villagers, from the houses around, joined the chase. He was not caught until he had run fifty meters on two broken legs. It took eight men and the doctor to drag him, still protesting that he was an airplane, back to the hospital. It took all eight to hold him down as the doctor set the fractures. The plaster casts were applied from the hip down to the toes. Immobilized by the casts, he thrashed his arms wildly about the bed until exhaustion finally conquered him.

Then, the grotesque and macabre parade began.

Mixed with those who were genuinely stricken with wild and uncontrollable psychoses were those who were victims of emotional hysteria, so great was the fear throughout the village. The hysterical would have to wait; the psychotics would require all the resources of the hospital and more. Not that the cases of purely emotional hysteria that developed would not require treatment under ordinary conditions. It was a question of emergency priority. A hasty "admission test" was arranged. Only those with clear-cut, now-classic, physiological symptoms were admitted. First, if they had *bradycardie*—the slow pulse, and *mydriase*—the enlarged pupils, the chances were they were the hopeless victims, and required containment. Second, if they were sweating and creating the odor of mice, a further confirmation could be made. For the problem now was the sheer physical matter of containment, treatment of any kind being ineffectual.

There were three strait jackets in the hospital. By shortly after midnight they were all in use. Nearly twenty strong male volunteers were called into service. The fire department surrounded the hospital. The police were massed in the hallways. It was a rear-guard action of retreat; the conquest of the disease was becoming more remote than ever.

They were nearly all screaming and shouting that long night, as they were brought into the hospital on stretchers, from trucks, cars, wagons, any form of transportation that could be pressed into use. There was the man and wife, both bleeding and disheveled, who had been chasing each other around the kitchen table with knives. There was the woman with delusions of grandeur, who insisted that she was a baroness and screamed that she was being persecuted when they dragged her through the hospital doors. There was the woman who was absolutely certain that her three children had been drawn and quartered and were hanging from the rafters of the attic to be made into sausages. There was the man who clutched his head because he was sure that red snakes were eating his brain. There was the man cringing and twisting his body in contortions because there were bandits with huge donkey ears chasing him. There was the seven-year-old child whose every toy changed suddenly into a fantastic, indescribable beast. There was the woman screaming that her son was dead, although he stood beside her and was helping her up the hospital stairs. There was the woman shouting, "You've come to kill me, to poison me!" There was the man who saw the hospital attendants as giant fish with gaping mouths, ready to eat him alive. There was the woman surrounded by the dead everywhere.

The delusions were not all horrifying. Some heard giant celestial choruses singing in the heavens above. Others saw flaming, gorgeous bouquets of flowers growing suddenly out of their hands and feet. Still others saw colors of the most breathtaking beauty everywhere, surrounding everything. Some saw in the most ordinary things—a thimble, a fingernail, a shoe—the whole essence of the world and the universe, a revelation they had never had before, a great religious mysticism.

But most were in terror. As one doctor approached a victim on her bed, she screamed: "No, Doctor. Do not approach me. Do not come near me! Look at the fire roaring from my fingers! *Regardez!* It roars out of each of my fingers. I do not want you to burn up! *Ne me touchez pas!*"

The attacks were fluctuating. The victims would come into sudden moments of perfect lucidity, recalling what had happened, but not understanding why they had seen such visions. Often, they were aware that the monsters and flames that they saw in front of them were not real, yet they saw them just the same. Actually, the moments of calm were as terrifying as the waves of psychosis, because the victim, in a fully rational state, would lie in desperate wait for the next attack to come, anticipating it, dreading it, knowing it was impossible to fend it off.

Outside the hospital, the shocked and stunned families and friends stood, looking up at the lighted windows, hearing the screams of those they loved, helpless to do anything for them, lost in confusion, wondering who among the watchers might suddenly become the same as those who were inside.

The strength, the violence, of the victims was almost unbelievable. At times it took up to fourteen men to hold one man down. With no more strait jackets available, the victims were lashed to their beds, screaming in horror. But the bonds would not hold. As the night continued, the load on the doctors, the sisters, the firemen, the *gendarmes* became overwhelming.

Victims were now breaking away from their bonds, running back out in the streets, and spilling into the hospital garden. There they uprooted tomato stakes and used them to fight each other; the firemen and police were forced to chase them, tackle them, and hold them down. By two in the morning they were holding, or attempting to hold, more than forty raving maniacs in the hospital, and the number was growing by the hour; the manpower to handle the impossible situation was growing proportionately smaller.

Knowing that the night shift on the Mondragon dam project was breaking, Dr. Gabbai requested the police to solicit volunteers from the workers there. Some fifty workers volunteered; they arrived just in time to help clear the hospital garden and help hold down the struggling victims when they broke away from their ineffectual bonds. The doctors, having gone almost two hundred hours without sleep, were coping with a situation in which medicine made no impact whatever. Haggard and drawn, they directed the volunteers to confine and contain in order to prevent utter self-destruction by the victims. The noise, the confusion, the stench, were indescribable.

Earlier, the doctors of Pont-Saint-Esprit had taken a few precious moments to call for more interns from Nîmes. But as the night progressed, it became evident that this was not a problem for doctors alone. The victims would have to be interned at the psychiatric hospitals in the nearest cities—Nîmes, Avignon, Montpellier—hospitals equipped for severely stricken psychiatric patients. At one in the morning the doctors reached the prefect of Gard at Nîmes by telephone and told him that the situation had now become so grave that upward of fifty people would have to be committed to asylums and that special ambulances to handle such patients must be dispatched at once. But the prefect's hands were tied: No person under law could be committed to an asylum without the preparation of elaborate commitment papers. On the average, it required almost three hours to fill out one paper for one patient. It would be an endless job of paperwork, requiring a skilled staff working at top speed. He did not have the authority to waive the ruling, which was strict, and clearly spelled out in the law.

In despair, Dr. Gabbai realized it would be impossible to handle the situation under such a restriction. He put a call through to the minister of health at Paris, and went back to the turmoil of the wards to wait for the call to go through. Numb from frustration and lack of sleep, he and the other doctors tried to improvise new ways for holding down the demented people—especially in view of the fact that a dominating symptom seemed to be commonplace: The desire to jump from the windows. One victim, just arriving at the hospital, required immediate medical services. Mme. Rieu, an elderly lady of the village had suddenly left the bedside of her equally sick husband, and plunged out the window of her home. Her fall was broken by a trellis, but her leg was fractured severely, and she joined M. Puche as a second victim of the insane suicidal desire to jump out the window.

Setting the fracture, the doctor's attention was drawn to a significant new sign: In addition to being severely ill, both of Mme. Rieu's feet were showing signs of gangrene.

In the middle of such chaos, a single symptom, even if serious, might go by without attention. But in addition to trying to save the affected limb, Dr. Gabbai's thoughts dwelt for the moment on the significance. Gangrene was a clear and specific symptom of historical ergotism, and along with the psychical outbreak, pointed toward a deductive confirmation of the growing feeling among the doctors that ergotism was the cause.

But there was no time now for anything but action. He set the leg, made the patient as comfortable as possible, and went back through the wards to supervise the groups of workers, police, and firemen as they held down the struggling victims by sheer force. A sudden commotion drew his attention in the corner of the ward, and he went toward it. Pushing through the crowd surrounding the bed of Joseph Puche, the aviator who thought he could fly without a plane, the doctor found the firemen holding back his arms as he strained to push them away with superhuman strength. He had been quiet only moments before, and had been left alone for a few moments while the firemen had turned their attention to others needing more care and restraint. Suddenly, someone had noticed that he was sitting up, and had literally ripped off half of one of his plaster casts with his bare hands. Before they could reach him, he had ripped off most of the rest of the cast, and was beginning to tear the other. Sick at heart, Dr. Gabbai began to cut off the remaining plaster in order to reset the fractures.

By three in the morning, now Saturday, the phone call came through to the minister of health in Paris. He assured Dr. Gabbai that the ruling would be waived, and that he had already ordered the prefect of Gard at Nîmes to immediately commit, on a temporary basis, all those who had need of emergency containment. By 4 A.M. the prefect had called the Hôtel-Dieu to say that help was on the way, including more *gendarmes*, militia, interns, strait jackets, known as *camisoles de force*, and ambulances.

Meanwhile, the holding action at the hospital continued. The patients, alternating between their moments of lucidity and hallucination, formed a continuous, undulating pattern that drew the volunteer workers back and forth across the wards to hold down those who had slipped their makeshift bonds and were desperately struggling to get to the windows. The compulsion to jump continued through the night. Guards were put at every window. One volunteer worker from the Mondragon project suddenly became stricken himself and had to be tied to a bed by his fellow volunteers.

The odor of mice and stale urine in the wards was overwhelming. The volunteers and hospital workers put handkerchiefs over their faces in a vain attempt to stave off the odor. A common vision among the sick was that of fireballs coming toward them, then receding and coming back again. *Zoopsie,* hallucinatory visions of animals, was rampant among the victims, as was logorrhea, excessive and incoherent talkativeness. Later, it was learned that the obsession with fire was what caused so many of the victims to want to jump out the windows. The sensation of imminent death and the delusions of persecution were also frequent all through the night. One fireman, taking a brief rest outside the hospital in the night air, told a bystander: "I hope God will never allow again what I have lived through this night." He was a veteran Resistance fighter who had been captured by the Nazis and had known all the full terror of the Occupation.

In their calmer periods the patients talked of the astonishing, brilliant, vivid, intense, and unbelievable colors—orange, red, brilliant white, moving in spirals, glowing from objects—that encompassed all their surroundings. Others described the conviction that they had been in a vast room, where the ceiling descended and the walls closed in on them, ready to crush them to death. Or there were those who described the feeling that their arms were pulling into their bodies, their knees telescoping up into their shoulders and chest. Auditory hallucinations—the noise of a clock, music, voices—were rare, but were noted by some. Three of the victims were absolutely sure they were witnessing their own funerals and actually invited the fatigued volunteers to take part in the obsequies. Nearly always the same hallucination returned to each individual, varying little from the one that struck the victim at the beginning. Some patients were in helpless confusion, knowing neither time nor space. Some were not even able to perceive heat when they were so tested. Often the tetanuslike convulsions would seize the patients and throw them into uncontrolled paroxysms, usually at the times the hallucinations began again.

As the doctors and the workers at the hospital fought their losing battle, the mayor and other red-eyed officials were at the town hall, attempting to coordinate transportation and essential information for the stricken and their families. The crisis was no longer a local one; it was now one for the *département* and for the national government itself. The one local ambulance was hopelessly inadequate; it would be considerable time before the reinforcements could arrive from Nîmes. All emergency phone calls were automatically routed to the mayor's office by the telephone company. When the voice of an anguished relative or friend pleaded for immediate assistance, the siren of the one local ambulance would scream again, with the piercing, undulating wail that only a French ambulance has. Ambulance sirens would start up 135 times in the next three days. A makeshift statistical system was organized. Short forms of commitment papers were improvised; names and addresses of the victims were recorded on a growing list that seemed to have no end.

As the overburdened and hopelessly inadequate ambulance reached the source of the latest call, the *gendarmes* and interns who had arrived from Nîmes after the first request would leap out, carrying the stretcher and an improvised strait jacket made of canvas. Neighbors, many in night clothes, would gather in the cramped alleys and hallways to see who the new victim was. Weeping relatives would follow the stretcher down the narrow stairways, vainly trying to comfort their loved ones. Other relatives would stand aside, pressed back against the ancient walls of the house, hands and fingers to their cheeks, in horror and despair. The struggle to hold the patient on the stretcher, even though he was strapped on it, was most often monumental. As the cortege passed, looking much like a funeral procession, neighbors would vainly try to comfort the frenzied relatives.

M. Guigou was taken from the Hôtel Redortier this way, as well as M. Rieu, who was to join his wife at the hospital, now lying prostrate with her leg in a cast, and gangrene in both feet. The condition of all three was most disturbing, showing the same signs revealed by M. Mison as he was taken to the hospital at Nîmes some days before.

The holding battle in the streets and the wards of the hospital went on until dawn. The ravishing beauty of the Provençal sunrise went unnoticed, though half the town was awake. It was market day, and the merchants, arriving from out of town to set up their stands, were greeted with the news of the tragedy that had struck the village. But life had to go on, and they began, tentatively, to assemble their wares and booths with the recognition that trading, if any that day, would be chaotic.

Their first direct experience of the extraordinary plight of the town happened shortly after their trucks and wagons had arrived. At dawn M. Sauvet, the garage-owner whose attack the day before had led him to believe that he was a strong man in the circus, stirred from the sleepless lethargy of his bed. His wife had left her own sickbed to go to the pharmacy, open all hours on emergency duty. Alone, he began to feel the inevitable signs of a new attack: the convulsive jerking of his limbs, the clouding of his vision, the stirrings of vague and ill-defined impulses which now filled him with dread. As he sank into his state, he summoned all his energies to combat it. He was fully conscious of what had happened before and of the remorse he felt afterward when he had surveyed the splintered bed and the ripped sheets. But gradually now, although he fought hard against himself, he again began to be convinced that he was a circus performer. He pushed the thought from his mind several times, but each time it returned stronger than ever. The combination of the rational and the irrational seemed to be tearing his consciousness to pieces. He was sinking into his delusion, and soon became aware that it was impossible to resist it. His bedroom on the rue Beauregard was assuming the proportions of a dressing room in a circus wagon before his resisting eyes. The walls were a lovely color, a rare and exotic color he had never seen before. His night clothes seemed to change miraculously into the tight-fitting leotards of a circus acrobat. Strength and confidence surged into him. Usually somewhat timid and afraid of heights because they caused him great vertigo, he was surprised at the feeling when it first began, but thought nothing more of it as he marched out his door, down to the Quai de Luynes, and along the embankment of the Rhône, his nightshirt swinging out behind him. For he was now an acrobat and a high-wire walker. There was no question in his mind.

When Mme. Sauvet returned from the pharmacy, she entered their apartment quietly in the hope that M. Sauvet had been able to find some sleep, which he needed so badly. All night long he had lain awake, despondent over his actions of the day before and pleading with her not to let it happen again. She came into the bedroom, saw the empty bed, and went immediately to the bathroom to find her husband. She rushed down the stairs to his shop, lying in disuse since the sickness had come to them. When she realized he was not there, she gasped and ran into the streets, shouting for help.

The neighbors gathered quickly, fanned out in several directions. M. Sauvet was spotted within minutes, far along the Quai de Luynes, approaching the bridge with a confident, swinging gait.

At the Pont-Saint-Esprit end of the bridge the last two arches had not yet been restored after the Allied bombing of 1944. In their place was a temporary suspension bridge, totally out of character with the ancient structure, but serving a useful purpose until the restoration could be completed. It was of conventional suspension-bridge design, with two temporary towers, from which hung the customary arc of the heavy cables supporting the smaller cables which held up the bridge floor.

Moments after he was first seen in the distance M. Sauvet began climbing up the side of the embankment by the bridge, near the fifteenth-century Maison du Roy. He moved swiftly and surely out onto the bridge, waving left and right in a magnificent and dramatic entrance into the circus tent that he alone could see. Before the crowd, including several merchants who left their stalls unattended, could reach him, he had already mounted the cable and begun a magnificent tightrope-walking act up the curve of the cable toward the tower. When the incline became too great, he dropped to his knees, and apelike, made his way halfway up the cable.

In minutes he was playing his high-wire act for a real audience: gaping villagers who watched him bow and acknowledge his imagined applause. Holding on with one hand, he would "style" himself in a grotesque arabesque high above the Rhône, which was directly below him, and the awed townspeople on the bridge and along the quay. In the crowd, Mme. Sauvet pleaded with him to come down, alternately covering her eyes and looking up again. Gingerly, two of the *gendarmes* made their way up the cable and gently tried to persuade M. Sauvet to come back down, but without success.

The high-wire act continued for almost fifteen minutes. Hastily mustered firemen, exhausted from their macabre night at the hospital, improvised a net extending out over the boiling Rhône. Gradually the pseudoacrobatics began to fade into jerky, uncoordinated movements. M. Sauvet swayed dizzily, then sat down on the cable, clenching the sides of it with both hands. He began inching slowly toward the outstretched arms of the *gendarmes.* The crowd stopped its murmuring, and a silence fell over it. Mme. Sauvet caught her breath, clutched the shoulder of a neighbor. The forms of the two policemen and the slight body of M. Sauvet grew closer together, inches at a time. He was now trembling and withered, no longer the brave and glorious acrobat. His shaking hand reached out for that of the first *gendarme*. At first they did not meet, and the crowd gasped as M. Sauvet lurched sideways. Then he regained his balance and lunged into the arms of the first policeman, the second one steadying the two of them as they inched further down the cable to the sidewalk of the bridge. Mme. Sauvet burst through the crowd, embraced her husband, and clung to him as he was guided to the police car. The crowd, in subdued horror, dispersed and made their way back toward the streets of the village.

By now it was just after six. At the hospital, the scene continued its undulating violence-and-relapse pattern. The exhausted staff would feel at times that the moments of calm were increasing, only to have an outburst explode in the corner of the ward, more intense than ever.

The convoy appeared on Route National 86, the main road from Nîmes to Pont-Saint-Esprit, crawling down the last hill from Bagnols-sur-Cèze, moments after M. Sauvet was led away to the police car and the Hôtel-Dieu. Later, it was described as "*une petite comédie de Provence.*" Right now, it was deadly serious. Leading the convoy was a Peugot 403, the automobile of the director of the hospital at Nîmes in charge of the expedition ordered by the prefect of Gard. Several members of the hospital staff accompanied him. Immediately behind was a military ambulance, with six attendants from the armed services as a crew. Its windows were ominously barred. Behind this was the psychiatric ambulance from the Nîmes hospital, with six white-suited interns. A third ambulance followed with six hospital orderlies from

Nîmes, also dressed spotlessly in white. Further behind was a car containing six Nîmes firemen in full uniform. The caravan wound along the route de Bagnols, past the home of Dr. Gabbai, reached the place de la République. Then it turned right at the corner, past the Fontaine de la Navigation, then down along the Boulevard Carnot to the entrance of the Hôtel-Dieu. Greeted by the Pont-Saint-Esprit doctors, the fresh, new staff moved into action immediately.

The worst cases, the most violent, were taken first. As the crews approached them in the wards, great confusion blossomed again. Untied from their beds, the victims fought with superhuman strength against the strangers from Nîmes; strait jackets flew across the wards as the victims tossed aside both crew and equipment in their struggle to free themselves. The reinforcement crews again were not enough. Merchants left their stands unattended to help. The patients were brought out the ornate doorway of the Hôtel-Dieu to the Boulevard Carnot, where the three ambulances were waiting. The uniforms of militia, police, national *gendarmes*, orderlies, interns, and firemen blended with the street clothes of the merchants and workers and the hospital gowns and torn remnants of the victims' clothing. Relatives and friends, trying to bring reassurance, struggled to get through the police lines, tears streaming down their faces. Pushed behind the barred windows of the vans, the victims continued their wild struggles inside, even though their arms were now restrained by the *camisoles de force*. Some of the relatives, victims of the milder and purely psychological hysteria, pressed their faces against the barred windows and beat on the sides of the vans in despair and frustration.

Officials made frenzied attempts to fill out commitment papers, even though the ruling was temporarily waived by the special dispensation from Paris. Authorities pleaded with relatives to sign the papers, but many were reluctant, fearing some vague kind of reprisals and reproaches from the victim when he was released. Adding to the chaos created by the genuinely psychotic was the collective hysteria in the village, which had mounted now to gargantuan proportions. The doctors insisted and checked that the precise physiological criteria be applied to all who were assigned to the Nîmes ambulances so that those suffering from the collective panic would not be confused with the others. No horror film could have created a more overwhelming scene. Orderlies who had been used to handling violent mental patients were stunned by the scene that greeted them. One of them commented that he would rather try to handle five demented persons trying to attack him than one who was trying to escape.

By now the core of reporters from Paris, Marseilles, Nice, Bordeaux, Switzerland, Spain, and Germany had grown to nearly a dozen. More were on the way. The doctors, the relatives, the authorities, even the patients, were harassed by them throughout the morning. They went to any length to take photographs, following the overworked and exhausted doctors, eventually throwing up a wall between the press and the townspeople, who united solidly against them.

Heartbroken through it all was M. Briand. His wife was in bed now, unable to move for several days. He had not been able to sleep for over two hundred hours, another victim himself of the same poisoning that had stricken everyone. He kept endlessly asking the same question in his mind: "Where did I go wrong? Where did I go wrong?" The words, the phrase, became an obsession, an *idée fixe* that matched the intensity of the compulsions of all the others who were stricken. He was, in a sense, a double victim: physically sick from the bread, emotionally shattered by the thought that his bread had brought mass tragedy to the village. Over and over again in his mind he retraced the night of August 15–16 and the processes he and his helper went through. The gray flour haunted him, yet it had been almost standard among all the bakers over the preceding weeks, and their protests had been loud. He was not a chemist, had no way of even dreaming that the flour could have been so deadly. And how could his bread *alone* have contained such a concentrated amount of whatever poison it was? What about the other sicknesses, just coming to public light now, from the bread of M. Jaussent, M. Monier, M. Griotti? His shop was clean; there were no other ingredients involved except flour, water, yeast, and salt. Why was the system of distribution so cumbersome that the bakers had to take what they were given from the Union Meunière? Why had something so unbelievably tragic happened to him after thirty years as a *boulanger*?

As the major outbreak raged through the town, M. Briand resolved that he himself would try to track down the cause, if there were any possible way he could do it. He knew that technically he was responsible for the results caused by what he delivered to his clients, but he would at least be able to search for the primary cause, and place the ultimate responsibility where it belonged.

His bitterness against the attitude of the Union Meunière was profound. In effect, all the bakers had been told by the organization: "The flour you are receiving is difficult to 'work,' but work it anyway."

He had "worked it anyway," as all the other bakers had done. The result was that he sat, impotent, and saw himself, his wife and his helper fall desperately ill, and his friends and neighbors become raving maniacs. His sorrow and confusion were overwhelming. As a deeply religious man, he prayed, but even that failed to bring him any comfort.

To punctuate his feeling of hopelessness that morning of the *crise*, a woman went by the shop, stopped abruptly, and spat on his window.

It took two round trips by the three emergency ambulances to clear most of the severe cases from the Hôtel-Dieu. The scenes, as the victims were forced into the barred vehicles, were heartbreaking. The doctors had not only been without sleep for over two hundred hours, but during the latest crisis, had not stopped to eat. Even with the arrival of the additional internes from Nîmes, they could not slow their efforts. There were decisions to be made about the cases, about who might remain at the Hôtel-Dieu, about where others were to be sent, diagnoses to be reported, relatives to be informed, temporary commitment papers to be organized and approved. In addition, new cases were coming. The local ambulance was continuously wailing out from in front of the Hôtel de Ville all during the morning. Ambulances were also arriving from Avignon, Orange, and Montpellier. These were put into local service or sent out to surrounding villages, or used to carry the victims to the most propitious hospital. The children were sent to Avignon; the most violent, to Montpellier and Nîmes. But no real classification could be set up under the chaotic circumstances. The main objective was to prevent people from destroying themselves until the disease could be pinpointed and some kind of therapy could be found that worked. The only consolation for some was that no more victims had died, although many felt this would have been less horrible than the terrifying, nightmarish scenes that continued during Saturday morning. That the victims had to be taken so far away from the village was most painful to the relatives, as was the appalling sight of their loved ones behind iron bars as they were driven away.

By noon Dr. Gabbai was able to turn his attention to an urgent message from La Villette. The farmhouse was a shambles, according to the messenger who brought the news. Mme. Testevin was helpless, and Emile, naked, was running amok in the yard, threatening to run into town. The other three patients were hopelessly psychotic in the upstairs rooms, though apparently under control.

Dr. Gabbai commandeered the military ambulance and its crew and led them out to La Villette in his own car. News had spread in the village that everyone at the farmhouse had died during the night, and when the doctor and ambulance arrived at La Villette, a crowd had gathered around the iron entrance gate, in spite of the fact that this was a considerable distance from the center of the village.

Emile was standing, naked, on the dung pile, shouting at the top of his lungs. Mme. Testevin was by the well, pleading with him to come into the house. Emile was yelling that he had to go to the barber shop, but couldn't because of the animals surrounding him. He cried out to Mme. Testevin to get the tigers out of the way, so he could go into town. Dr. Gabbai came in through the gate and walked directly to Emile. He had great respect for the doctor, and the entrance had a major effect on him. His voice died down from a shout, and more softly he begged the doctor to get the animals out of the way.

The doctor played along with his delusion, softly persuading him to come down off the pile, and move into the house. He did so, reluctantly at first, more cooperatively later. In the house he slumped on a chair in the wrecked confusion of the dining room, weak, listless, silent.

Calling in two of the military aides from the ambulance to watch Emile, the doctor went upstairs to look at the other patients with Mme. Testevin. Her husband was resting quietly on the bed, shouting out instructions to his hunting dog. In a sudden change of scene, he invited the doctor to join him in a meal which he believed to be in front of his eyes: Giant pheasants and thrushes, crisply roasted and garnished with rich sauces, a huge vat of *potage de légumes*, a tub of *salade Niçoise*, a side of *bifteck* drenched in gravy. This Pantagruelian feast, the doctor surmised, was a reflection of the frustration M. Testevin faced from the restrictions placed on his diet over the past years because of his liver condition. Two other victims had demonstrated the same delusions the night before; each of them had been on carefully regulated diets before the outbreak.

Madame Dezeuzes was still crying, not having stopped the entire night. M. Delacquis, conscious of the doctor's entrance into his room, was back in bed, and introduced eight of his army companions from World War I, who he insisted were sitting in a circle around his bed.

Coming out into the hall, the doctor said, "Emile must be taken away. It is urgent."

"But he needs our care," said Mme. Testevin. "The hospital will make him worse."

"He is very sick. All of them are very sick. But he is the worst. You cannot possibly handle all this."

Mme. Testevin was adamant. "It will make him worse. He is quiet now, isn't he?"

"It will not last long," said the doctor. "They will stay quiet only for moments, then go off again."

"I'm sure I can make him well again," she insisted.

"Would you rather have me send your husband?" The doctor was firm.

"Will they take good care of him?" she asked.

"They will do everything they can," he said. "There are so many like this. You must understand."

There were four strait jackets in the ambulance. They brought two of them in, for in some cases during the previous night one strait jacket had been ripped by the violence and extraordinary strength of the victim, a feat difficult to accomplish even under severe strain. Two orderlies and two of the military aides approached him gingerly from both sides, because the doctor had warned them about Emile's strength. Quietly but ready for any emergency, they took hold of each of his arms. Emile rose meekly.

They wrapped a blanket around him and led him out through the yard, past the staring crowd.

Mme. Testevin, watching from the doorway, was crying, but she was also tense. What would they do if Emile, with his enormous strength, fought against going? She watched as they led him out through the gate and up the back steps of the barred van. Inside, she could see them strap his arms down to his sides. He was still passive. He did not resist. She noticed a large pair of handcuffs dangling from the back pocket of one of the orderlies and the two strait jackets over the arm of another. Emile was staring straight ahead, apparently not conscious of anything around him.

"Please, God," she muttered to herself, "don't let them have to use those things on Emile."

The doors of the van were closed, and it began pulling away. Emile had gone quietly, and her prayer had seemed to be answered.

But the wagon had gone only a few feet when she heard from within it a muffled shriek of the most blood-curdling intensity. She clutched at the arm of Dr. Gabbai beside her, and turned her head away.

SEVEN

When the caravan arrived on its first trip to the Centre Hôpital of Nîmes, the crews led, pulled, tugged, and lifted the patients from the barred ambulances into the psychiatric wing, where extra beds had been hastily erected. Directing the operation was Dr. Georges Pitot, who with his thick lenses, cropped hair, and long white jacket, appeared calm and organized in spite of the chaotic scene in the open driveway of the hospital. Spectators were gathered here, too, watching from the driveway entrance in impersonal awe. There were no friends or relatives now, no tears, no outcries from the spectators.

Emile did not remain quiet.

Seven of the crew tried in vain to drag him from the ambulance, while the other patients in his ambulance threw themselves against the walls and seats, trying to climb over and out of the door to the illusion of freedom.

The shouts all around from the patients continued without cease.

"Why are you bringing me here? Why? Why? Why?" a victim who had returned to his senses was crying. "I am well again.

Please, please, please, don't put me in here. Not behind bars, please! I have done nothing wrong!"

Beside him, an older man was crying, "My belly is full of snails. They are burning me to death! I am in the water. I am sending out radio messages everywhere. Get me the X ray, get me the X ray, and you can see!"

A woman in the same ambulance beside him, waited her turn quietly, her head lowered. "My son is dead, my son is dead," she kept repeating.

Another, a young man, was crying, "Please, Sirs, cut my skin. Cut my skin! I'll feel better. Get me a bicycle and cut my skin!"

But Emile, the last to be removed from the ambulance, was saying nothing. He was fighting—fighting with a fury that held off the seven men and the reinforcements sent to aid them. Sweating, grim, determined, two of the crew at last slipped a strait jacket over his arms. They shouted with relief to the other orderlies outside the van. But then they watched in stunned amazement as Emile ripped the tough canvas and split it down the middle with his hands. Another *camisole de force* was passed along. Incredibly, he ripped that one also. The orderlies were replaced by the military aides, with more strait jackets in reserve. They worked and struggled, as Emile tore through seven consecutive strait jackets. Finally they were able to envelop him in two strait jackets at once, and the battle was over.

Scuffling, kicking, he was dragged out across the driveway and up to his cell with its barred windows, its tiny observation window in the iron door, its irrevocable lock. With the same detachment that all who work with the demented must assume, the orderlies tied him to his cot with giant leather straps as he strained against his strait jackets. The crew left, locked the door, and went back to their gruesome and unwelcome job of bringing the others to the same fate.

Emile, his arms and legs bound with leather, had a moment of lucidity as he lay there on the cot. He desperately wanted his freedom, but all he could do was stare at the ceiling. Various memories—the giant, grotesque animals; the tigers; the fight against phantasmagoria; the shattered furniture in the dining room; the scene on the dung pile where he stood naked and had the insane desire to go to the barber shop—passed through his mind. He kept asking himself why he had done these things. Why did he see those animals, at once so real and so illusory? Why was he suffering so? What had happened to his mind, his emotions, and his feelings? He was a kind man, a man who loved people, who loved his work in the vineyards with the rich soil, the smell of grapes, and the tying of the vines. He cried when he thought of what he must have done to Mme. Testevin when she tried to help him during his attack. He loved the Testevins and was almost a member of the family. They treated him with love and kindness, and he worked on the vineyards as if they were his own.

Then a veil began descending over his consciousness again. The straps were biting at his arms and legs. He must get back to La Villette to make amends for his utterly destructive actions. He must tell Dr. Gabbai how sorry he was to have caused him so much trouble. He must explain why he acted the way he did. The tigers had been so real he had felt their breath on him; he had felt the wetness of their giant mouths and the sharpness of their teeth; that they had been real and not-real at the same time; that the colors of the walls and of the trees and of the dung pile had been so vivid they made a rainbow into a dwarf of dullness; that he must repair the furniture, straighten the room, return to his work with the harvest time coming so near. He must do all this; he must not lie here in this cell any longer. He must act, and act at once, because though he hated it, he could see now, clearly and unmistakably, another tiger in the corner of the room. He was licking his paw, casually, indifferently, taking occasional glances in Emile's direction. Emile lifted his head to look at him. Now he was confused. Was the tiger real—or imagined? He could no longer doubt its existence. And why was it staring at him now? Why was it rising, stretching, breathing more heavily? And why was it coming toward him now, slowly, threateningly, directly to him until its eyes were now enormous, its mouth slobbering right by his throat.

He shrieked. The echoes in the empty room thundered back at him. Then the tiger pounced toward his throat. No one paid attention to his screams, because there were others doing the same thing in their cells all along the corridor.

Sure that the tiger was now engulfing him, he bent his head down toward his right arm, found that his teeth could reach the thick leather strap. Frantically, he began chewing, sinking his teeth deeper and deeper into the bitter, thick and sweat-soaked leather. He chewed and ripped away chunks of the strap as wide as the palm of his hand. Spitting them out, he attacked the strap again, until his jaws ached and he felt excruciating pain in his teeth. He began to taste blood. He spit out another large chunk of leather—and with it, two of his front teeth. Now he worked with the side of his mouth; slowly the strap gave way, and one hand was free. He attacked another strap, and more of his teeth fell out on his chest. There were more animals coming into the cell now from every direction: giant spiders, snakes, more tigers. Desperately, almost sitting upright now, he continued eating his way through the second strap. More of his teeth fell out on the floor and the bed until all the top and bottom teeth in the front of his mouth were nothing but stubs or roots. Then he pulled himself free of his fixed bed and rushed to the barred windows. Turning, he saw the horrified face of an orderly in the tiny observation window. The man called down the corridor for help.

They were all coming to kill him now, Emile felt. He gripped two of the iron bars on the window, pulled them in a frenzy with every ounce of strength he could summon. They moved, bent nearly an inch under his superhuman pressure. The blood in his mouth was filling his throat; his teeth were splitting with pain.

He was slumping by the bent bars of the window when the six orderlies burst into the room. It took all of them to grapple with him, skid him down the hall, down the stairs to a subterranean cell.

Dr. Georges Pitot, psychiatric chief of the Centre Hôpital de Nîmes, took a great deal of pride in his growing psychiatric section of the hospital. Born in 1904, he had taken his medical training at the University of Montpellier, and his psychiatric specialization at Marseilles. Now he and his wife, Dr. Marguerite Pitot, were in the process of rebuilding the psychiatric staff and equipment at Nîmes after the severe disruption of the Second World War.

Like Dr. Gabbai, he had been on vacation when the tragedy first struck Pont-Saint-Esprit. Driving back in two days from the Alps, he arrived to find M. Mison at the hospital in the throes of death, but the extent of the sickness was still not clear. Everybody who could be of possible use was being mobilized, and being a systematic man, he began the attempt to analyze the symptoms, while the toxicologists were desperately trying to organize the analysis of the bread samples and viscera.

Along with the other doctors, his feelings leaned toward the ergot theory as the most possible cause; but like the other medical men, he was working in the dark, and he was cautious. The most detailed case histories of outbreaks of ergot poisoning were from the seventeenth century, and in researching them he found that the descriptions were far more literary than scientific. Two days before the night of the crisis at Pont-Saint-Esprit, "the night of the Apocalypse," he had pored over the ancient papers and read of the plagues of ergotism that had struck several mid-European villages in times past. He found that the doctors then had fought the outbreaks of St. Anthony's Fire, or *mal des ardents*, with the same futility the doctors in and around Pont-Saint-Esprit were facing now.

"This disease is caused by the usage of bread and of flour containing ergot of rye," he read in the *Dictionnaire Encyclopédie de Science Médecine*. It was a musty volume, with yellowed pages and a cracked cover, published in 1887 in Paris, and unearthed now in the medical library at Montpellier, where Professor Gaston Giraud, dean of the School of Medicine, and Professor Hughes Latour the *chef de Clinique* were already at work correlating their own personal observations with the information coming from the doctors at Pont-Saint-Esprit. "Linne [a French physician of the time] gives it the name of Raphania"; the text continued, "Wepfner [another doctor of the epoch], that of *Convulsio ab ustilagine*; others, that of *Convulsio cerealis*. The common names are St. Anthony's Fires, malignant fever, and convulsion of Sologne [a region of France]."

The tract went on to say that this disease had raged in epidemic form in Silesia, Prussia, Bohemia, Sweden, and in some of the provinces in the center of France, particularly in Sologne. Among the most severe epidemics were those in Württemberg in 1735, Gatinais in 1674, and Lucerne, Bern, and Zurich in the same general era.

The epidemics, it was noted in the text, seemed to occur after years of considerable rainfall and were due mainly to the negligence of the farmers, who permitted ergot-diseased grain to be mixed in with the ordinary grain, creating an inferior, disagreeable flour. The year 1951, the doctor reflected, had been wet and humid. The dictionary went on to say that there were many doubts as to the origins, the etiology, of ergotism, and it was thought that perhaps the general low level of hygiene experienced in past epochs contributed to the outbreak of the disease. One doctor attributed the mysterious and elusive cause to the seeds of a plant known as *Raphania raphanistrum,* mixed with wheat and rye. There was no doubt, however, that the Fire of St. Anthony was due to ergot, regardless of the mysteries concerning its exact properties.

The symptoms, the encyclopedia explained, consisted of dizziness, stupefaction, and extreme troubles of the sight and hearing. A sort of drunkenness developed, and in many cases, severe convulsions. With the convulsions was great delirium, and the pupils of the eyes dilated widely. There was gangrene of the extremities in some cases. Furthermore, during the epidemics of the seventeenth and eighteenth centuries the victims suffered severe heartburn, a feeling that they were alternately burning up and freezing, and a loss of the consciousness of time and place, in addition to the convulsions and the extreme hallucinations. Not all who died suffered from gangrene, but all the victims generally showed a slowing of the pulse and circulation.

Also noticed were severe damage to the eyes, severe digestive upsets, and hemorrhages experienced by women, along with some cases of abortion. But, the paper concluded confidently, all of this is only of historical interest, since "the epidemics of St. Anthony's Fire are no longer seen. . . ."

Dr. Pitot noted with a grim irony that the seventeenth-century treatment for the disease, reviewed by the doctors of 1887, included bleeding, emetics, purgatives, and tonics. Opium and ammoniacs had also been used. This was hardly very helpful advice in the face of all the present-day sick in Pont-Saint-Esprit. The fact was that even modern medical research offered little or no hope for constructive treatment against the diseases of ergotism. The most advanced treatment merely withdrew the source of the poison and alleviated the symptoms: maintaining adequate circulation to the extremities; using vasodilators such as choline esters, nitrites, and papaverine; relieving nausea and vomiting with atropine; and prescribing calcium gluconate for muscle pains unresponsive to massage and exercise. Again, hardly effective ammunition for fighting dozens of raving maniacs and scores of others unable to sleep for nearly two hundred hours, even if indeed the ergot theory were correct.

The other historical material available to the doctors was hardly more comforting or illuminating. There were the pictures of the flaming indignities provoked by St. Anthony's Fire during the Middle Ages. In 1089, an observer wrote: "We could see many 'ergotists' in the village, bowels devoured by sacred fire, either dying wretchedly or living with gangrened limbs." When the town of La Motte-au-Bois in the province of Dauphiné, some hundred kilometers from Pont-Saint-Esprit, was stricken by ergotism in the Middle Ages, a nobleman and his son, both afflicted with the disease, called on St. Anthony and were cured by what they thought was the presence of St. Anthony's relics in the town. The relics had been captured by the Saracens in 532 and taken to Constantinople, but they had been brought back to Dauphiné by a conscientious pilgrim. The nobleman and his son then set up a lay society to cure the ill who were smitten by the disease. Even then the disease was nothing new. Ergot in rye had been mentioned in the Bible by the prophet Amos; Pliny had mentioned it in his *Natural History*. It was used in the tenth century in Thuringia for its strange power to hasten childbirth; it is still used under controlled modern medicine for the same thing today. "There is a tingling and burning of the hands and feet," one writer described the symptoms, "and then a frightful heartburn. Fingers and toes are bent nearly double and clamped; the mouth is full of foam. Often the tongue is lacerated by the strength of the convulsions. There is a severe secretion of spittle. The sick utter that they are being destroyed by a burning fire. They feel great giddiness, and some of them become blind; the intellectual capacities are polluted, a fog comes over and destroys the mind."

The more sophisticated observations of the nineteenth century recognized that ergot was a parasitic fungus growth on grain, called *Claviceps purpurea*. A dense tissue forms in the ovaries of rye and gradually replaces the entire substance of the grain with a hard, purple, curved body called the sclerotium. This is the commercial source for pharmaceutical ergot, recognized in modern medicine as a very useful but often puzzling drug. It was only in the nineteen-thirties that many of the ergot alkaloids were discovered and defined chemically, but even today many facts are elusive. One thing is certain: All the ergot alkaloids are derivatives of lysergic acid, a chemical that still has much mystery surrounding it today. Useful for migraine, epilepsy, hypertension, hastening childbirth, and other diseases, the ergot alkaloids, improperly used, are dangerous.

The many signs in the historical and medical material that pointed to ergotism as the cause of the Pont-Saint-Esprit tragedy still proved nothing. There were certainly close historical parallels here, but Dr. Pitot knew that modern medicine could not proceed totally on hunches and that the most pressing current necessity was the research of the toxicologists, who were now working with a formidable mass of specimens that had to be carefully handled or the tests would be next to useless. In the meantime, as the ambulances screeched into Nîmes with their flailing, writhing human cargoes, Dr. Pitot recognized that he and his colleagues faced a major embarrassment. Tranquilizers in the postwar France of 1951 were unavailable, and there was no indication that they would be effective if they were available. Such barbiturates as gardenal and morphine were useless, as were the hypnotic drugs, which are usually very effective in curbing psychotic outbreaks. The lamentable and tragic fact that had to be faced at the moment was that the doctors had no other therapy for all these suddenly psychotic people, who were usually perfectly normal, but strait jackets and leather straps.

The shrill cries of the ambulances in the village of Pont-Saint-Esprit did not stop all through the following day and night. The calls were less frequent now, but the uncertainty about when and where the next blow would fall continued to hang like a pall over the town. The villagers struggled to carry on their ordinary, everyday affairs, as if by sheer force of will and attention to the concrete details of existence, they could erase the memories of the previous nights. It was a hopeless attempt, of course, because the crisis was still continuing. The Eynards both went to their office the following morning, and oddly enough, found that none of their patients had canceled their dental appointments for the day. M. Boudenne opened up his hat-and-sporting-goods store as usual and sold several new fishing rods, a large rubber beach ball, a new set of *boules,* and two pairs of tennis shoes. Mme. Carle, still weak and utterly despairing about little Marie-Joseph, who was now tied to her bed in the hospital at Avignon, found that she could stop herself from a complete breakdown only by checking the inventory at the grocery store; her husband, in the bedroom upstairs, continued to boom out the numbers of the window panes—one through six—without stopping.

Mme. Eynard found that she could keep her mind in better peace by helping her husband and trying to concentrate on examining molars and bicuspids, although her mind kept slipping back to the scenes of horror they had witnessed the past two days. Their office was directly beside the Hôtel de Ville, outside of which the ambulances with their barred windows stood, mutely waiting for their next call. Each time the sirens wooshed into action, she felt as if their building trembled and winced at the thought of the scenes that would be taking place as the back doors of the vehicles were swung open, and another victim was whisked away from his weeping relatives and neighbors. She listened to many stories from the patients that morning; a persistent one being that many of the victims had now escaped from the hospitals and were coming back to wreak vengeance on their relatives for permitting them to be taken away. One of her patients, who had seemed perfectly normal, left the office and suddenly started to scream in the streets beside the ambulance outside the town hall. She was swiftly led into the ambulance and taken away.

Leaving the office at lunchtime, the Eynards encountered two friends, a husband and wife, and they talked quietly about the urgency of the situation and what could be done about it. The couple was concerned because they had eaten a considerable amount of the bread; they had already been ill, but were feeling better that day. By nightfall they had been taken away to Montpellier, both demented. The young engineer joined the Eynards for lunch. When he volunteered to go out to buy matches, which they needed, he found himself carrying several potatoes from their kitchen with him. Word from Francine was that her sister was still sitting at the kitchen table, never sleeping, never speaking to anyone, and in almost complete catatonic withdrawal. The worst shock to Mme. Eynard was seeing formerly normal men and women suddenly change and then seeing their contorted faces—sometimes hopeless, sometimes protesting, sometimes beseeching—staring out the barred windows of the ambulances.

The reporters—now nearly thirty of them—were sweeping over the town, continuing in greater force their demands for information, which even the authorities could not give them. They congregated at the Café de l'Univers, the Café des Voyageurs, the Café de la Bourse, sipping *pastis* or vermouth, trading information, making macabre jokes, sliding a few francs to waitresses and bartenders for fragments of information. Where information was lacking, creative ingenuity came into play. One reporter bought a mess of fish, took them to the Rhône, and threw them in, along with some large chunks of bread. He photographed the dead fish swirling in the current by the bread, and sent the picture back to his paper in Paris with the caption that even the fish had been poisoned by *le pain maudit*, "the accursed bread," as it was now labeled by another enterprising reporter. The phrase caught on and has remained the label for the entire tragedy over the years.

The Paris headlines screamed with the news: THE POPULATION OF PONT-SAINT-ESPRIT NO LONGER DARES TO EAT BREAD . . . MONSTERS AND FLAMES HAUNT THE MINDS OF THE POISONED OF SAINT-ESPRIT . . . TERROR AND MADNESS HANG OVER PONT-SAINT-ESPRIT; THE MYSTERIOUS "ST. ANTHONY'S FIRE"? In French, the impact was stinging: TERREUR ET LA FOLIE PLANENT SUR PONT-SAINT-ESPRIT; FEU DE ST. ANTOINE?

"It is neither Shakespeare nor Edgar Poe," wrote one reporter.

> It is, alas, the sad reality all around Pont-Saint-Esprit and its environs, where terrifying scenes of hallucinations are taking place. They are scenes taken straight out of the Middle Ages, scenes of horror and pathos, full of sinister shadows. The doctors are beside themselves with work; the rumors are wild and contradictory; fear hangs over the village everywhere. No one knows when it will end.

A terrifying new rumor was gaining, a rumor that seized the village with the most excruciating terror. It was passed from mouth to mouth with a most electrifying speed. A wild and insane criminal was loose in the town, had poured poison into the flour, and was now at work poisoning the water supply and all the food of the merchants he could get his hands on; he was so subtle and diabolic that he masqueraded as a respectable person; no one would know who he was by observing his actions. He appeared so normal he could be anybody's friend or relation. When the police took into custody an unnamed man for questioning, the rumor was fanned into a blazing bonfire. The more timid of the population boarded themselves in their houses, drank Badoit, Vichy, or Evian water, and prayed that they would not be stricken themselves.

At Bagnols-sur-Cèze, M. Gillot, an inspector in the antifraud squad, *inspecteur au Service de la Répression des Fraudes,* was pawing through and minutely examining three hundred empty flour sacks that had been placed under seal by his department. Somewhere in the forest of sackcloth might be the clue that could unravel the mystery, which was becoming more horrifying every day because it lurked so deeply in the shadows of the unknown. As M. Gillot counted away in the thick white dust of the warehouse, Commissioner Georges Sigaud questioned Jean Bousquet, the forty-five-year-old distributor for the Union Meunière, about the flour that had come into the region under the distribution system. What *wagons* had arrived at the station at Bagnols-sur-Cèze since the first part of August? Where had they come from? Were they sealed properly? What were the numbers and dates on their labels? How many kilograms came from what millers? What deliveries had he made to M. Briand? To M. Jaussent? When, and under what circumstances? How were the sacks transported? In what trucks? How many quintals of flour came from M. Maillet? How many times had M. Bousquet demanded that the Union Meunière do something about the gray flour being delivered? What did he tell the mayor of Saint-Génies-de-Comolas when he protested so loudly about the flour? It was a long, tough interview. But it was not a question of hostility. Each man was as anxious to find the common enemy as was the other.

Since August 23, the press had been promising that the results of the laboratory tests would be immediately forthcoming. These predictions, however, failed to take into account the complexities of the job faced by the toxicologists, The authorities and the police were swamped with demands for a definitive answer to the cause of the poisoning, and this led them in turn to place more pressure on the laboratory in Marseilles. The pressure was useless, since the toxicological results were controlled by chemical processes and reactions that simply could not be hurried.

The bread samples that were collected by the Fourteenth Mobile Brigade and sent to Professor Ollivier at the police scientific laboratory at Marseilles were tagged and labeled as to their sources, carefully wrapped, and ready for processing. Some of them were full loaves from M. Briand's shelves; others were half-eaten loaves or chunks and crumbs that had been gathered from the kitchens of the villagers. Samples of flour scooped from the sacks in M. Briand's bakery and in other bakeries were also sent. All of these items had to be submitted to tests that demanded both classic and specific techniques: the former to obtain a general, over-all picture of the constituents of the material, the latter to pinpoint specific constituents which were suspected. The two techniques differed, required dividing the sample, whether it was viscera, bread, or flour, and submitting it to prescribed tests that sometimes required days.

One test for alkaloids of ergot was conducted by a process known as the *réaction de Keller*. It sought for and determined the amount of lysergic acid present in the specimen, since lysergic acid was the base of ergot. To accomplish this, Professor Ollivier would place the specimen in a tube, and evaporate a portion of *l'éther alcalin*, and then add to this residue 0.2 cubic centimeters of a dilute solution of a chloride of iron and cooled acetic acid. Then 0.2 cubic centimeters of pure sulfuric acid would be allowed to trickle along the wall of the tube, until the two liquids met. The presence of alkaloids of ergot would then be indicated by a blue ring that forms, and diffuses in the liquid on agitation. An additional test, the *technique d'Hofmann* would then be applied, in which the bread would be pulverized dry, then ether and sulfuric acid added to form a liqueur, which afterward would be submitted to a centrifuge. Present-day tests, however, are considered more accurate.

In addition to the search for lysergic acid, the tests were continued for the possibility of traces of arsenic, antimony, bismuth, barium, copper, zinc, thallium. There were also other possibilities to search for: mescaline, hashish, poisonous fungi, opium, even marihuana. In turn, there were the tests to determine the power of the toxicity by injecting or feeding samples to mice or guinea pigs. With the eyes of the French public and press on him, Professor Ollivier was determined not to reach a hasty or incorrect conclusion that could be more dangerous than none at all. He was harassed by the necessity of interrupting his laboratory work to journey to Montpellier for the autopsy of M. Mison.

Not that the professor was without his critics. Some felt that he did not have the experience to handle a complex case of this sort, in spite of his numerous titles on the faculty of the University of Marseilles. One critic pointed out that he had never been placed on the list of experts of the Tribunal at Marseilles, even as a toxicologist, chemist, or biologist. Some felt that his pride prevented him from seeking outside help when he needed it. Regardless of his critics, he was working around the clock, exhausted and as anxious to reach a solution as the police, the press, and the public.

Commissioner Sigaud, as much at the mercy of press and public pressures as Ollivier, continued bulldozing through the endless job of turning up clues, whether they were criminal or accidental in nature. The criminal theory was alternately pursued and discounted. To the horror of the villagers, it could not be overlooked. There was always the gnawing possibility that the poison might not be actually related to the flour. M. Briand was interrogated several times, at extreme length, as well as his helper, who, though more ill than M. Briand, was able to get up from his bed now. Every detail of the night of August 16 was reviewed several times by Commissioner Sigaud. What time did his helper borrow the flour from M. Jaussent? How many kilograms of his own flour did he have on hand before he mixed it with the flour he borrowed? Did both he and his helper prepare the *pouliche,* the preliminary mixture, before the definitive *pâté*? Who did the weighing of the dough, the balling of it, the shaping? What was the appearance of the sack of flour borrowed from M. Fallavet? Was that flour gray in color too? When did Mme. Briand begin to feel sick? Himself? What kind of seal or label were on each different sack involved? It was a slow process, an overwhelming one in the face of the mass of details that had to be collated and analyzed. And as M. Sigaud investigated, interrogated, and unwound a mass of clues and evidence in the Midi, the Mobile Brigade in the north, in Poitiers in Saint-Martin-la-Rivière, where the flour had originated, pushed its inquiry under the same pressures. The public and the journals wanted more than a knowledge of the cause; they wanted blood. A report from the north was expected momentarily. Commissioner Sigaud hoped that a clear break would come from that direction to take some of the load off his overworked shoulders.

With the shipment of new flour into the village, the bakeries reopened. Once again the townspeople could be seen with the long, unwrapped loaves under their arms, strapped to bicycles, or poking out of shopping bags. M. Briand began again, with sorrow, but with the resolve that he must go on in the face of the tragedy while he conducted his own bitter inquiry into its cause. Many townspeople rallied to him and demonstrated their faith and confidence by buying bread as they always had. Others were sullen and vindictive. One woman, seeing him across Grande Rue, dropped her shopping bag in the street, went into hysterics, and hurled a steady stream of abuse at him. Sadly, he turned away, slipped behind the door of his shop, and tried to continue his routine as well as he could. In spite of the loyal clients, his trade fell off markedly. He counted the leftover loaves at the end the first day after the reopening: More than half had not been sold.

In a statement to the press M. Briand tried to clarify the tragic circumstances of the baking of the bread on the night *le pain maudit* was made. "I am convinced," he said, "that the poisonous bread came from the second lot of bread baked that night. There is proof of it in a particularly tragic fact: I forgot to make my usual delivery to one of my clients in Carsan, M. Mison. He came into my shop to reproach me. I gave him then two loaves from this baking. A few days later he was dead."

Later, he told another reporter: "I've been a baker here for thirty years. You don't suddenly poison your clients after all that time. A bakery isn't a laboratory; all we have is salt, yeast, and flour—and maybe some margarine for pastries. There is nothing foreign in the shop that can get into bread and poison people. I use no drugs or flavoring. But every man has to accept the tragedy that comes his way. This was not something I sought. It was fate that struck me after thirty years. Being a baker is hard work, most of it at night—long, hot, and difficult. I always use the same salt, the same yeast, the same water. Only the flour changes, and I must accept what the Union Meunière gives me. My bread was poisoned, but why? Why especially has it killed only one man, whereas others are still living?"

Mayor Hebrard, without sleep for nearly seven days, also made a statement to the press. His slight frame was slumped; his eyes, red-rimmed. "I have seen sane beings suddenly become seized with terror, horror and fury, ripping their sheets or their curtains, cowering and cringing to escape the hallucinations. Charles Pommier, a dear friend of mine, barricaded his door and armed himself with his shotgun to save himself from the monsters that were pursuing him. Joseph Puche jumped from a high window. Four of the townspeople have attempted suicide. Many have tried to jump from the windows. It is truly a nightmare that has come to our village."

The nightmare was unrelenting. As he talked, the ambulance, sirens wailing, was streaking to some remote corner of the village, and another victim was added to the growing list. It totaled now just a few less than three hundred, not increasing as much in quantity as in the seriousness of the cases that had once seemed to be improving. One villager, for instance, had been doing splendidly. His digestive troubles had cleared up, and his alternate sweating and shivering had stopped; only his insomnia remained, but that was so common that it had become accepted by both the stricken and the unaffected. It was cases like this that gave people comfort; there seemed to be an end in sight. That was why it was all the more tragic when this same man, crossing the Boulevard Gambetta and nodding happily to a friend, suddenly ran screaming past the office of the Eynards and into the police station, where he demanded to be arrested or put out of his misery, since, he screeched, both his arms and legs were on fire.

More unrest came to the townspeople when they heard that a hunter just outside of Pont-Saint-Esprit had to shoot his dog; it had suddenly gone mad, its fur standing on end, and attacked him. The stories filtering back from Avignon were particularly horrifying: Lovely small children shrieking for their mothers, tied day and night to their beds as they pitifully tried to rip their bonds away. The rumor that a criminally insane maniac was responsible for all the tragedy persisted. Only the absence of further fatalities prevented the panic in the streets from becoming overwhelming. Without further deaths, there was greater hope.

This faint hope did not last for long. As his wife was taken from the Hôtel-Dieu to the hospital in Montpellier, her leg encased in its bulky plaster cast, Paul Rieu was removed from his home to the same place, his convulsions and hallucinations now combined with a cardiovascular collapse. The two lay in the same room at Montpellier, but neither was conscious or rational enough to know that the other was there. The condition of both was most disturbing; they showed the same symptoms as had M. Mison when he had been taken to the hospital at Nîmes some days before. M. Rieu, seventy-two years old, died first, in convulsions. Within two hours his wife, with severe gangrene of the extremities, joined him in death.

There are stages of exhaustion in times of utter chaos and duress when the human mind cannot absorb all the shock forced on it. The news of the death of the Rieus was received in stunned silence, as if the people were saying, "What else do you want of us? You have taken our loved ones away in strait jackets; we have watched them try to tear themselves apart—and now, this. Who of us is to be next?"

The headlines caught the atmosphere of the town, as only a French newspaper could: THE POISONED BREAD: A SECOND AND A THIRD DIE AT PONT-SAINT-ESPRIT WHERE 50 MALADES BECOME SUDDENLY AND FURIOUSLY INSANE . . . ARE THEY VICTIMS OF A SORCERER'S HERB OR OF AN ODIOUS CRIMINAL?

The New York Times, less vivid, but measurably more outgoing than usual, headlined the story: THREE DIE, MANY STRICKEN BY MADNESS FROM POISON IN BREAD IN FRANCE.

Meetings were almost continuous at the Hôtel de Ville. Professor Giraud, along with Professor Latour from Montpellier, and Professor Recordier from Marseilles, conferred in secret with the local doctors, then went out on personal rounds of the patients in the village. They overlapped the visits of the Bishop of Nîmes, Msgr. Girbeau, and the Canon, M. le Chanoine Jullian, as they tried to bring comfort and renewed faith to the sick. They saw, both doctors and religious men, the scenes that had been going on ever since the full fury of the epidemic had struck. They heard the spasmodic wails of the ambulances, still continuing. They saw M. Carle, who ignored their presence, lying in bed, monotonously counting the window panes, droning the numbers one through six, then beginning again and again without cease. They saw Mme. Charpail sitting at her kitchen table, eyes on the floor, responding to neither her surroundings nor her guests. They saw Mme. Briand, bed-ridden and weeping from her illness and her sorrow for what their bread had caused. They saw M. Sauvet, quiet now, and rational, filled with apprehension that he might be overcome by his strange compulsion again.

At La Villette they saw M. Testevin, lying still in the semidarkness, still talking of the hunt, the chase, and the Pantagruelian feasts. They saw Madame Dezeuzes sobbing without let up, thin and drawn. They saw M. Delacquis, his fingers almost raw from writing, knees propped up, barely acknowledging their visits.

M. Delacquis had another visitor that day, Mlle. Wullschleger. She had closed the office early for the lunch hour, walked out to the *mas* in the hot noontime sun, hoping that she would find some improvement in her *patron*. He was in a period of lucidity when she came into the room, although he could not stop his compulsion to write. He had great pain in one eye, he told her. He still saw the huge balls of fire come toward him at night—and also the visits of his World War I companions. He summoned the energy to ask about the office work, but his worry about it grew, and Mlle. Wullschleger changed the subject. She was shocked at his appearance, "thin as a skeleton," she put it. She knew by now that nothing could make him stop writing. He grew wild and frenzied when he could not write. She brought him, as usual, some new pads and sharpened pencils, and she tidied up the old sheets as she gave him the new writing equipment.

What M. Delacquis did not tell her was that whenever, in his lucid moments, he found himself without a pad and paper, he would stare at the window, then feel inevitably drawn toward it. He would feel almost a gravitational force pulling him with such strength that he gripped the side of the bed to stop himself. He knew that if he reached the window, he would jump. There was no question in his mind. It came mostly at night. He would seize the pad and pencil, write furiously of his thoughts, his phantasies, his dreams, anything to get his mind off the window and the window sill.

But the verses, the songs, the prose that he wrote brought him freedom from the compulsion. And that is why he felt he could not stop. He did not write senselessly. Even in the moments when he was not related to his environment, his writing was precise, his verse disciplined. Mlle. Wullschleger picked up a sheet one time to read, although afraid that she was invading his privacy.

It was a poem, simple, direct, poignant:

Dark hours—ashes
That fall and cover up
All the things, and the soul.

Dark hours—opaque vapor
That comes up from the bottom of everything
And fatally like an ebb
Invades the voids of life.

Dark hours—monotonous song
In a minor key, sad and full of torture;
Rhythmic sting of the dagger
Into the mass of brain.

Dark hours—acid taste
That makes the mouth grin
The whole tragedy of life,
The dark hours.

There were others, too, and she was touched by their poignancy:

Man the unknown who is just beside me,
You have a face so full of goodness.
And your eyes are so clear
Before you sink into somber nothingness.
I would like to read one page of your life.

Where do you come from? Where do your steps go?
What thoughts trouble your mind?

What fervent desires remain unspoken,
Shake so strongly under the edge of your skin?

Do you suffer the vile lashes of anxiety?
Are you the lover of an insatiable chimera?
Do you, like me, cry on the beautiful summer days,
Raising your eyes toward the unfathomable skies?

Has the pack haunted you unkindly?
Are you a prisoner of a circle of impatient,
Sinister dowsers of anguish?
Is your heart filled with triumphant love?

Man the unknown who is just beside me,
I would like to read a page from your life
Because I feel you are my brother.

There were tears in the eyes of Mlle. Wullschleger when she left La Villette that day. Why should such a sensitive, creative and considerate man lie in a bed alternating between sanity and psychosis, living in an obscurity that showed no promise of lifting? And when would it stop? At La Villette and all through the town? As she walked down the hill, toward the red roofs of the village, the wail of another siren split the quiet midday silence.

Although the news about young Joseph from the hospital was good, Mme. Moulin was still too ill to go and see either her husband or son. Her daughter, a young *pharmacienne* living in Lyon, had arrived. But she was most often away from the house visiting her father and her brother, supervising the transfer of them from Villeneuve-les-Avignon to Nîmes, when a serious crisis arose. Young Joseph, alternating between apparent recovery and relapse, had gone into a coma after a fit of hallucinations and convulsions, alarming the staff at Villeneuve-les-Avignon, who were not equipped to handle such serious cases. After they were moved to Nîmes, both father and son seemed to be making extraordinarily good headway. Heartsick with both husband and son in the hospital, Mme. Moulin continued her battle against the constantly reappearing doctor in the dark suit and the "head of death." Each time he suddenly appeared in the kitchen doorway, with the black staring eye sockets, the noseless face, the jawbone hanging loosely on its hinges, she would scream at it and tell it to go away. She would throw anything she could find at it, knowing the futility of such an act, knowing that the figure was nonexistent. One afternoon her brother-in-law arrived just after she had been yelling at the apparition.

"What is wrong, my sister?" he said. "Has the sickness returned stronger to you?"

Aware of her own folly, she quickly recovered her composure. "No, no there is nothing the matter," she said. "It is only the dog. I was yelling at him. He has been naughty."

She constantly found herself doing this, covering up her sickness when visitors came. She tried desperately to reason with herself, to rid herself of the grotesque vision, but could not prevent it. "I must pull myself together," she would mutter to herself, but in the stillness of the house, the *tête de mort* would reappear, and the cycle would begin again.

In Nîmes young Joseph was in good spirits.

For one of the few times since he had been brought to the hospital at Nîmes, he was able to sit. Even the moans he heard from the neighboring rooms, the macabre shouts of his fellow patients in their undulating periods of hallucinations, could be borne better, now that he felt some of his strength returning.

Up to this moment, the prognosis had been gloomy. For days, tied to his hospital bed, he had been crying monotonously: "There is a stone on my heart! Please lift it off, please!" The news of his worsening condition had leaked back to his mother, struggling with her own phantoms at home. She had often lied to her neighbors, saying that she had received a letter from her son telling her how well he was getting. At one time young Joseph had risen weakly from his bed, moved to the door, and looked out the observation window. Across the hall, he had watched, horror-stricken, as a woman victim of *le pain moudit* had flung herself around her cell, tumbling, rolling, and jumping, singing wildly as she did so, literally tearing her hair from its roots. This, he was sure, was what he was like when the convulsions and hallucinations struck him, so unpredictably, so frequently. But this day was different. There was even news that his father was improving. Mayor Hebrard, visiting all the sick of his village interned in the

Montpellier and Nîmes hospitals, stopped by to see him, chatted aimiably with him.

"Your mother is improving greatly at home, Joseph," said the mayor. "And the work in the vineyards is going along well, even though they miss you." Mayor Hebrard knew he was stretching the truth, but felt justified.

"I am so glad to hear that," said Joseph. "And to hear the good news about my mother. I hope she'll be able to come and see me soon. It has been a terrible struggle. For all of us."

They talked for a few more moments; the mayor excused himself and left. A little later, young Joseph's sister arrived and was delighted with his progress. Perhaps the wide, dark curtain of despair was now going to lift after such a long *entr'acte*. Convinced that the crisis was over, she left to return to help her mother back at the *domaine*.

It was not long after she left that young Joseph felt again the icy, physical heaviness in his heart. He fought against it, tried to hold it back. Then the convulsions came, and with them, the hallucinations.

By midnight young Joseph was in a coma. At four in the morning, Wednesday, August 29, he died.

EIGHT

A SMALL EDITORIAL item in *le Midi-Libre* ("*Grand quotidien d'information du Midi*") had been read, reread, and quoted by many *Spiritpontains* as a source of comfort during the days of chaos. It said: "The poison, whatever it is, acts seriously only on those who are aged, rather than on young people, probably because the young are able to eliminate the poison better."

Young Joseph Moulin was twenty-five, strong and hearty. The news of his death, compounded by the double death of the Rieus, brought a new surge of panic through the town. Moreover, people were still running amok in the streets, several days after the terrifying night of mass madness. The feeling of distrust of friends and neighbors still prevailed everywhere. Some actually avoided chance encounters in the street, feeling that perhaps the acquaintance to whom they were talking might insanely rush at them without warning.

The double funeral of M. and Mme. Rieu punctuated the grimness of the atmosphere. The shops in the village closed their doors as the two caskets moved through the narrow streets, out to the walled cemetery on the road to Carsan. A large, somber, and silent group gathered by the graveside, the hot afternoon sun broiling the black-clothed mourners. Mayor Hebrard read a solemn tribute to the couple, revered and loved in both the town and the surrounding countryside. He demanded that justice be sought and gained, whatever the circumstances turned out to be. At the ceremonies were General de Philip, *conseiller général* of the canton of Pont-Saint-Esprit, sweltering in his uniform and Sam Brown belt, and the mayor of the neighboring town of Bagnols-sur-Cèze. It was not a funeral in the ordinary sense, because all who stood beside the two coffins, as they were lowered into the double grave, felt deeply the distinct possibility that the next services could be for their loved ones—or even themselves.

A new meeting that night at the Hôtel de Ville brought together the prefect of Gard, M. Batailion, *directeur du Service Départemental de Santé,* General de Philip, and the three exhausted doctors of the village. At the conclusion the prefect made an official announcement that was unable to satisfy the craving of the populace for firm and uncloudy information.

"While waiting for the conclusions of the *expertise,*" the announcement read, "which cannot be known for at least two or three days from now, the tentative conclusion of the doctors who have treated and studied the cases is that the poison is a question of a vegetable alkaloid, creating a convulsive reaction on the vascular system.

"The judicial inquiry in the northern provinces—in the *départements* of Indre and Vienne—will reveal if there has been negligence or shortcoming at the source of the flour delivered for the bread made in Pont-Saint-Esprit."

The statement, necessarily vague and indecisive, infuriated the victims and their families, and brought forth vociferous demands for clarification. Among the doctors, both from the village and from the universities, there was a division of opinion. Lacking laboratory confirmation, Dr. Vieu, Dr. Gabbai, Professor Giraud, Professor Latour, and Dr. Pitot were inclined toward the ergot theory. The symptoms were now beginning to coincide more and more with the classic ones for the disease, but all the doctors were intelligent enough to withhold final opinion until all the results were in.

Dr. Channac, on his part, was inclined to disagree. "It is, in effect," he said, "strange that the poisoned flour has been delivered only to a single bakery in Pont-Saint-Esprit."

Overlooking, or not being aware of, the sicknesses in the area that had presaged the major outbreak at Pont-Saint-Esprit, he went on to say: "Because of the modern methods that the millers employ in preparing the flour, the entire region and all the bakeries would have been affected. But the cases of Pont-Saint-Esprit seem to have come from a *single* sack of flour, in which the poison seems to have been concentrated. Is it not possible that this sack had been placed in contact with an insecticide or some other toxic chemical?"

His question was apt and bore serious consideration, as did many other postulates that were developing, aside from the accusations of poison gas, the English, the Pope, Stalin, and bacteriological warfare. The criminal-maniac theory persisted, but no basis for it could be found. M. Briand delved deeply into background material in his own research. He read of sicknesses in ancient Palestine and Egypt from a grain called *l'ivraie,* which had been mixed with good grain and had caused convulsions, hallucinations, and nervous crises similar to those caused by ergot. He studied the reactions of those who had taken peyote or the sacred mushrooms of the Mexican Indians, many of which were the same as the reactions of the victims of Pont-Saint-Esprit. Professor Euzières, a member of the faculty of the School of Medicine at the University of Montpellier and a psychiatric specialist, found similarities of symptoms with persons poisoned by an herb called *Lathyrus sativus,* otherwise known as *gesse commune.* The ingestion of this herb had created paralysis and mental derangement.

Professor Ollivier, again interrupted in his laboratory work to go to Montpellier for the autopsies of M. and Mme. Rieu, conferred with his staff before he left and surveyed the inconclusive results to date. Many preliminary tests had been concluded. The pressures to release some kind of official information had now grown to the point where the safety valve seemed ready to let go. He felt it would be wrong to release the incomplete information he had on hand. At Montpellier reporters badgered him for some kind of statement, and attempting to hold them off, he said:

"The analyses are extremely long and delicate, especially in view of the fact that all the samples sent to the laboratory are not toxic. It is necessary to submit them to some processes that require observation for four or five days. The tests on the guinea pigs often demonstrate that some samples are not poisonous. If the samples do turn out to have adverse effects, it is then necessary to examine the animals' tissues and their viscera—another time-consuming process."

Over the protests of the reporters he left them to join the other doctors in their autopsy of the second and third victims to succumb to the mysterious malady.

They went about their work in the somber gloom of the Montpellier Hospital with the detachment from tragedy that only medical men can have. Somewhere in the muscles, the brain, the duodenum, the intestines, the heart, the glands, or the blood were clues that could lead to the solution of the mystery.

In the blood it was necessary to look for carbon dioxide and to study the hemoglobin by utilizing spectroscopic techniques. They looked for evidence of hypnotic drugs, chloral hydrates, or ethyl and methyl alcohols. In the viscera, they sought evidence of chloroform derivatives, bromides, or phenols and other volatile poisons. They searched for the mineral poisons—phosphorous, arsenic, antimony, mercury, barium, bismuth, zinc, copper—as well as the nitrites, oxalates, fluorines, chlorates, and sulfonamides. The poisons of vegetable origin—glucosides, digitalis, and organic poisons—demanded special attention in view of the nature of the suspected origin of the yet unknown poison. The search for each toxic alkaloid demanded specific attention: atropine, heroin, nicotine, codeine, quinine, cocaine, strychnine, morphine, ergot, and ergot alkaloids, as well as hashish, peyote, and others. The job was gargantuan; it was a maze of delicate analytical complexities.

The results could not possibly be known in a day, nor in several days. Yet the pressures continued to build, and tension began to replace the methodical calm so necessary in the laboratory.

Pending more definitive results of the autopsy, Professor Ollivier returned to Marseilles, a gruelling three-hour drive. Here, the tests were continuing on the flour and the bread samples—piles of white dust, crumbs, chunks, crusty loaves—some of which still looked as tempting as the day they were baked. Still plaguing the research was the insufficient bulk in some critical specimens—insufficient for both the classic and special tests required for full clarification. In the laboratory at Marseilles, the mice, the guinea pigs, the rabbits, and the frogs sat mutely in their cages, awaiting either the fate of the victims of Pont-Saint-Esprit, or escape from it, depending on the specimen they received intravenously or by mouth. With the inanimate specimens, the tests were continuing in the same manner. This search for volatile, mineral, vegetable, or synthetic poisons was a race against time which was important not only because of the demand by the doctors, the police, and the public to know; but because the poisons could be chemically deteriorating under the eyes of the technician, under the lens of the microscope, or in the test tubes.

Reluctantly, Dr. Ollivier agreed that a progress report should be made public at this time, and he sat down to prepare it. The ordinances from the examining magistrate had been battering his office at a machine-gun rate. In one official order, M. Perrier had ordered the doctor "to proceed to research and determine if there are poisons or toxins or lesions provoked by any such toxic agents in the viscera of Félix Mison, and to determine the nature of his sickness and the cause of death." He further requested that Ollivier "analyze the flour or yeast seized." The judge noted that the dogs, cats, and ducks had been killed or poisoned by the bread, and added: ". . . to orient your research, you will be able to be in touch with the doctors who were called to take care of the sick who were poisoned. It is possible that any toxic substance could be of an organic nature; certain doctors have mentioned ergot of rye or wheat from parasitic rye. . . . I permit myself to give you this information only as an indication, and I ask you another time to hasten the completion of these tests, which are of vital interest not only for justice, but equally to the administrative authorities and the health department."

Later, Judge Perrier wrote again, instructing Ollivier to proceed with the autopsy of M. and Mme. Rieu to find out the cause of death, and he added: ". . . if you see fit, you should seek assistance from any and all competent specialists."

Dr. Ollivier did not see fit to bring in other specialists at this time, which later was to become an abrasive point with his critics.

On August 29, still another ordinance arrived, accompanying the samples of the bread of the Moulin family that had been baked on the morning of August 16. In addition, a sample from the bread baked by M. Jaussent was included as a control comparison that might have far-reaching effect on the case. "I am sending you," wrote the judge, "some bread bought at the Jaussent bakery. . . . If the Jaussent bread is toxic, we will be able to renounce with certitude the incrimination of M. Briand and orient our further research toward the distributor and the miller of the flour."

Dr. Ollivier was aware of the risks that a temporary statement might bring with it. But it seemed to him to be the lesser of two evils. The evidence, though incomplete, was there: Traces of ergot had clearly been found. On August 30, 1951, while the victims were still sporadically and suddenly going beserk in the streets of Pont-Saint-Esprit, while the ambulances stood silently in wait on the Boulevard Gambetta in front of the town hall, and while three other victims lay in unpredictable comas, Dr. Ollivier completed his summary in the form of a telegram to M. Perrier in Nîmes. If he had known the consequences that were to follow, he might never have sent it. It read:

MINISTERE DE L'INTERIEUR
TELEGRAMME
ARRIVEE

Transmission

Mention de service	*Origine*	*N⁰ Expedition*	*Numéro de Mots*	*Date et houre de depot*
	Marseilles	8337	89	12:55 30/8/51

EN EXECUTION VOTRE ORDONNANCE DU 21-8-51 J'AI L'HONNEUR PORTER A VOTRE CONNAISSANCE LES PREMIER RESULTATS POSITIFS DE NOS RECHERCHES STOP LES ECHANTILLONS DE PAINS MISON ET PAIN MOULIN DU 16/8 ET DANS LES VISCERES DU CADAVRE MISON FELIX D'UNE SUBSTANCE PRESENTANT LES CARACTERES D'IDENTIFICATION TOXICOLOGIQUE ET BIOLOGIQUE DES ALCALOIDES DE L'ERGOT PARASITE DES CEREALES STOP RESULTATS QUI SONT EN PARFAITE CORRESPONDANCE AVEC LES MANIFESTIONS CLINIQUES AT LES LESIONS AUTOPSIQUES PRESENTEES PAR LES MALADES INTOXIQUES ET LES ANIMAUX TEST STOP FIN SIGNE OLLIVIER

EXPEDITEUR—LABORATOIRE INTERREGIONAL DE POLICE SCIENTIFI-

QUE DE MARSEILLES A MONSIEUR PERRIER–JUGE D'INSTRUCTION–AU TRIBUNAL DE PREMIERE INSTANCE–PALAIS DE JUSTICE–NIMES–GARD

In fullfilling your ordinance of August 21, the telegram said, I have the honor to bring to your attention the first positive results of our research. The bread of the Mison and Moulin (samples) of August 16, and that in the viscera of Félix Mison presenting the characteristic toxicological and biological identification of the alkaloids of ergot, parasite of cereals. The results are in perfect correspondence with the clinical manifestations and autopsy lesions presented by the poisoned *malades* and the animal tests. End. (signed) Ollivier.

The telegram, like a giant rudder, was to swing the police investigation harder to the north, to the *département* of Vienne. Commissioner Sigaud, moving from Nîmes, Montpellier, and Pont-Saint-Esprit was in daily touch with the northern province, where the Seventeenth Mobile Brigade was at work tracking down every possible source of the grain and flour. M. Sigaud's police report—incomplete and pro tem also—had been filed immediately on the completion of the preliminary investigation before Professor Ollivier's telegram had been sent. The commissioner's report read:

"In the absence of the results of the analyses of the specimens of flour and bread which were seized, we are able to envisage three hypotheses:

"(a) The toxic agent was an alkaloid of vegetable origin coming from *ergot de seigle;* in this case it is necessary to trace the origin of the wheat.

"(b) The toxic agent was of mineral origin. It is then necessary to discover if the wheat or the flour had been placed in contact accidentally, whether in a silo, a mill, whether in the course of transportation, with toxic products utilized in agriculture.

"(c) The toxic was also able to contaminate the flour in the course of transport while traveling on the *chemin de fer.*"

When Professeur Ollivier's telegram arrived at Nîmes, its effect was electrical. In Pont-Saint-Esprit the news struck like a giant comber. Every dictionary available was opened to the word *ergot,* although the information was slight—hardly more than an indication that the substance was a parasite of certain grains and cereals, especially rye; a fungus growth, purplish in color. Some of the less abridged dictionaries indicated that it had been responsible for the plagues of St. Anthony's Fire, Holy Fire, or *mal des ardents*, and even indicated that its base was lysergic acid. Whatever deficiencies existed in the dictionaries were compensated for by the press, which burst out of its orgy of speculation, and flooded its pages with information on ergot. C'EST L'ERGOT DE SEIGLE! the headlines screamed, elaborating them with grotesque and sinister histories of the towns stricken *en plein moyen âge*. While the news stories did nothing to ease the raw and serrated nerves of the populace, there was almost a feeling of relief throughout the town. The enemy was at least recognized and spotted, even if the victims, who were being rushed to Nîmes, Avignon, or Montpellier more sporadically now by the ubiquitous, toad-faced Citroën ambulances, were still increasing.

Writing in *France-Soir*, Professeur Claude Moreau, phytopathologist of the Museum of Natural History in Paris, expounded on the mysteries of ergot for the puzzled minds of the laymen. He explained, somewhat patronizingly, that this fungus destroyed the ovaries of the grain, substituting a hard, black or purplish "*sclérite*," replacing the normal grain. It comes as a result of improper drying of the wheat, after a wet, damp growing season (which 1951 adequately displayed). The *claviceps purpurea*—the technical name of the parasite—attacks numerous wild and cultivated grasses, although rye is especially vulnerable. In very small quantities, the substance was not dangerous, but certain climactic conditions could produce many different kinds of ergot, and could create the rare affliction of historical ergotism. In addition to the Middle Ages plagues, parts of Finland were stricken in 1862. In 1926 an epidemic had hit Russia, in some regions striking 50 percent of the population.

A major problem with ergot is that it is unpredictable in potency and biological action, and presents mammoth analytical difficulties as well. There still remain many mysteries about it. Identified by modern science at the time—1951—were fourteen different kinds of alkaloids and thirteen amines.

Treatment was practically futile. Its ravages created the brusque contractions, the inhibition of the terminals of the sympathetic nervous systems. The extremities tingled and seemed to catch fire, the body trembled, there were spasmodic contractions, cramps, and sometimes gangrene. Skin rashes and severe hemorrhages in women often appeared. Heartburn, hallucinations, and the delusion of being on fire were often noted.

The intensity of the affliction depended on the quantity of alkaloids present, but these were illusive and frequently short-lived.

Articles in the press like this were small comfort to the villagers. *Banal* treatment—that of attempting to treat the symptoms alone, to replace inadequate nutrition by vitamins, to protect the patients from their own furies—was all the doctors had to work with, if indeed, ergotism turned out to be confirmed by further tests; there was no cure. Meanwhile, the insomnia of the victims was total, absolutely total, and created its own problems even among those who were not so seriously stricken. For those who suffered from an *idée fixe,* this was most torturing. They could not stop their compulsive absurdities, even though they were perfectly aware of how ridiculous these were. M. Carle finally found that he could check his interminable and loud counting of the six window panes, but only by substituting another *idée fixe.* He invented a word, "saxophile," and kept repeating it in a loud voice, *ad nauseam,* day and night, without stop. Another victim went into tantrums unless his children marched kettle tops on the kitchen table like soldiers. The family was forced to take shifts to satisfy this insatiable demand.

In all the chaos there were no sexual manifestations evident, no attempts at rape, no sexual phantasies or hallucinations. There were mystical revelations of a sort, vivid colors, and the strange euphoria, but specific sexual impulses were neither stimulated nor experienced. There were the badly stricken, who fought their hallucinations and convulsions in the hospitals and some of whom hung in a coma between life and death. There were those who were struggling at home to stop waves of psychotic feelings that swept over them unpredictably. There were the compulsives. And there were those who simply could not sleep, who ached for the day when they would be able to close their eyes and sink back in repose, a condition that by now had lost all meaning for them.

Commissioner Sigaud, the active arm of the examining magistrate, wrote in his notes on receiving the news of Dr. Ollivier's telegram: ". . . we have been advised that the first results of the toxicological tests have attributed the poisonings to alkaloids of a plant origin and derivatives of grain ergot. Our inquiry is now concerned more than ever with the first hypothesis we envisaged."

At Poitiers, some three hundred miles to the north of Pont-Saint-Esprit, Commissioner Sigaud went to join M. Gillot, fraud investigator at Nîmes, and M. Gagnier, who performed the same function for the region of Poitiers. It was from this region that the French National Railroad had brought the shipments of flour from the mill of Maurice Maillet to Bagnols-sur-Cèze, resulting in the protests of the bakers all around Pont-Saint-Esprit.

As the inquiry was closing in on him, M. Maillet told the press: "They cannot reproach me for anything. Never at any mill has there been the least negligence in making the flour. The flour I processed in June came from old grain, but if the flour coming from my mill has been delivered in a spoiled condition, I know nothing of it. The people responsible would be the transporters and the distribution organization in the département du Gard."

At three thirty in the afternoon of August 30, a police car arrived at M. Maillet's mill to take him and his assistant, M. Bertrand, to the Commissariat Central de Poitiers for further questioning. Commissioner Sigaud had already visited the mill and found it wanting. Maillet, a diminutive and sad-faced man in his forties, wearing a beret, was nervous and afraid. A taciturn man, he was the father of three children and lived quietly in Saint-Martin-la-Rivière, where he was well liked by his 1,200 fellow townsmen. M. Bertrand, his helper, was older by five years and struggled to keep his family of nine children in proper and respectable care. In contrast to the broad-shouldered, smooth-haired Commissioner Sigaud, intent and determined to solve the case with all haste, they presented a limp and pathetic picture.

M. Maillet's mill in Saint-Martin-la-Rivière presented an equally unimpressive appearance. It was old, having been run for years by his father before him, but the machinery for the milling was in reasonably good order, although it had not been replaced since 1932. The process of transforming the grain into flour here, as elsewhere, was completely automatic. The coarse wheat was blown into the mill, forty-five quintals at a time, falling automatically into a cleaning process that included a magnetic device to lift out the particles and slivers of metal accumulated in the threshing process. Then it was cleaned again by an apparatus combining ventilators, aspirators, and agitators. The milling, sifting, and grinding processes continued without interruption for forty-eight hours, until the flour was jettisoned into the sacks provided by the Union Meunière.

The exact shipments of flour from Maillet's *moulin* were quickly determined as the questioning began. Speaking with characteristic reticence and apathy, M. Maillet told the investigators that all the flour he had exported to the Pont-Saint-Esprit area by way of the distribution center of Bagnols-sur-Cèze was made exclusively of grain from his neighboring cooperative at Saint-Julien-l'Ars. He had, he added, made a simple addition of 1 to 2 percent of flour derived from beans, which is a customary, and perfectly legal practice. He insisted, however, that he did not add any secondary cereals, especially rye. This was a critical point, for ergot in quantity would be more likely to come from rye than wheat. Not satisfied with this answer alone, Sigaud immediately sent his investigators to check the cooperative and determine just how much grain they had delivered to Maillet. The register showed that 360 quintals had been sent to Maillet, but Maillet's own register indicated that he had received only 210 quintals, 150 less than the records of the cooperative indicated.

There was also a record of his having delivered approximately ten quintals of flour to a local baker by the name of Guy Bruère. This, Maillet told the investigators, was also a common practice. A baker would bring in his own grain to be milled so he would not have to purchase flour on the open market. The grain brought in by M. Bruère, M. Maillet explained, had not been mixed in with the grain from the cooperative. Maillet had processed it exclusively for the local baker.

"Why," asked Sigaud, "was this flour not put in the general mixture from the cooperative?"

"Because," Maillet answered quietly, "M. Bruère wanted to have flour from only his own grain. He preferred it."

Only a fraction of the flour from Maillet's mill had been shipped to local bakers. Maillet's helper, M. Bertrand, confirmed this when his turn for questioning came. But Sigaud was stopped short when Bertrand said that M. Bruère had delivered grain to the mill that he wanted to exchange for flour made from other grain.

"It was very bad quality," said Bertrand. "All of us noticed it. Bruère himself admitted it. The wheat was full of rye. But Bruère insisted that we take it and give him some of the good flour in return for it. He wanted the flour made from the grain of the cooperative. M. Maillet protested, but M. Bruère kept insisting. Then M. Maillet said, 'How do you expect me to give you good flour with the slops you are giving me?' Because there was not only a lot of rye in the grain, there were also moths and dust. M. Maillet finally told me that we had to work it anyway and mix it in with the grain from the cooperative. So M. Bruère took the flour already in the mill, and his grain was mixed in with the rest."

Sigaud, finding now a major discrepancy, began pressing harder. He brought in M. Bruère immediately and continued the questioning, while Maillet and Bertrand waited outside.

M. Bruère, dark, lean, and artistic looking, was in the process of taking over the management of a shop from another baker at Saint-Martin-la-Riviére. Like Maillet, he was a quiet and unassuming man, well liked in the community, and of sound reputation. He had arrived at the mill of M. Maillet with his load of grain on July 8, and he admitted to Sigaud that Bertrand had remarked on its bad quality—that it not only contained a noticeable amount of rye, but that it also included a considerable smattering of moths and dust. He also admitted that far from wanting flour made from his own grain, he had asked Maillet to give him some of the good flour in exchange. But he hastened to elaborate on this for the commissioner. "It is a current practice in our region to accept at the end of the season some grain of bad quality, mixed with secondary grain, coming from the bottoms of the silos." He also indicated that his accounting practices in skirting around the special legislation controlling the quality wheats and flours were kept in an "absolutely fantastic" manner. He pointed out, for instance, that the three farmers from whom he was supposed to have received the grain were nonexistent and he had collected the grain in small quantities from farmers who had traded him these scraps of grain for loaves of bread. He never actually verified the contents of the sacks. He was aware that all such transactions required legal permits, but he had never bothered to conform with the regulations.

In a brief respite during the questioning, the commissioner took the time to make a statement to the press. "By tomorrow morning," he said confidently, "we will truly know all the facts. I will make known all the results of my inquiry after the examining magistrate has reviewed all the depositions."

When M. Maillet was called back before the commissioner, his nervousness had increased. He had no idea whatever what information either Bertrand or Bruère had given Sigaud, but this did not remain a mystery to him for long.

"You have told us," said Sigaud bluntly, "that M. Bruère insisted on getting back flour from his own grain—that none of his grain was mixed in with that of the cooperative. Are you still convinced of the truth of that statement?"

Maillet hesitated, then spoke. "I have lied to you up to now. Actually, I gave Bruère the flour made from the grain from the cooperative. It was already in the process of being milled at the time. The grain he gave me was mixed in with the grain that was shipped down as flour to Bagnols. When M. Bruère brought me the sacks of grain on July 8, I noticed that many of the sacks contained a large amount of rye; others just contained wheat alone. It was then the end of the season, and the farmers were scraping the bottoms of the silos. When they were short of wheat, they filled in the rest with rye. I commented to Bruère about the condition of the grain he was bringing me. He told me that certain of his clients had owed him money and that he had accepted the rye in place of the wheat. He kept insisting that I work the grain for him. 'Give me less,' he said, 'if you wish, but give me something a little more palatable.' I accepted, and I replaced his sacks with the good flour from the cooperative. I honestly thought that the rye mixed in with a large quantity of wheat would be imperceptible and wouldn't cause the flour to be bad. My worker Bertrand knows everything that took place."

He paused a moment, then continued. "I know that at the end of the season the rye collected in the bottoms of the silos is of bad quality. I did not believe, however, that it would be toxic and dangerous, since I had seen flour of both wheat and rye mixed together during the war. I had accepted the mixture of wheat and rye because I knew that the farmers' quotas would be difficult to make this year. I knew nothing about ergot of rye and did not know how to tell the difference between that and normal rye. Neither did my worker Bertrand."

M. Maillet was relieved to get everything off his chest, and he continued. "All the bakers near me in our region are very particular about the quality of the flour they receive. They will accept only the pure white flour, and they refuse it when it is anything less. That is why I sent the flour containing the rye to the Gard, to Bagnols, for I feared the bakers in my region would cause me great difficulty in accepting it." (Later, Commissioner Sigaud wrote in his notes: "Evidently the bakers of the Bagnols and Pont-Saint-Esprit regions had less luck than those living near Maillet in Vienne: In spite of all their multiple complaints—which never resulted in any action—they were never allowed to refuse this flour in the manner that Maillet himself had done for the bakers of Saint-Martin-la-Rivière!!")

For the first time since the back-breaking investigation had begun, Sigaud began to feel that he was making progress. Here was a classic case of concealment. Maillet had denied mixing the more-than-questionable grain of Bruère. Bruère and Bertrand had revealed the facts. The bad grain had been dumped into the batch from the cooperative; Bruère had happily gone off with a few less kilos of good flour, but good flour nonetheless. For it, he had traded bad grain that would be part of the mélange shipped off to Bagnols-sur-Cèze and would later end up somewhere in the ovens of the bakers in Pont-Saint-Esprit.

In a preliminary telegram to the examining magistrate in Nîmes, Commissioner Sigaud wired the information that he and his investigators had definitely confirmed that the flour delivered to Pont-Saint-Esprit had come from Maillet's mill, that the mill appeared badly managed, that a sack containing waste and scraps from the flour made over several months before had been seized, and that he had found considerable rye in the scraps.

The questioning of Maillet and Bertrand continued through the night. Each shipment of grain and wheat was traced with infinite care. The stories were checked and rechecked with Bruère. By two-thirty the following afternoon the commissioner was able to sum up the entire results of his inquiry in another wire to the examining magistrate: Maillet and Bertrand had admitted accepting grain containing a high proportion of rye of bad quality as well as mites and dust; Bruère not only admitted this, but had declared that he had falsified his accounts in order to mask the fraudulent exchange.

On September 1, 1951, the formal charges were prepared against both M. Maillet and M. Bruère. They were indicted on four counts: (1) *Fraude alimentaire*, for supplying food that was uneatable and dangerous to public health; (2) infractions of the special legislation regarding flour, such as transporting and holding bread flour in containers other than sealed sacks, lack of special registration of the flour, and sale and purchase of flour containing a high proportion of secondary cereals; (3) infraction of the special legislation regarding wheat and grains, including the lack of proper records of the shipment and receipt of the stocks; (4) involuntary homicide and injuries.

In the early evening Bruère and Maillet were arrested.

Commissioner Sigaud, now reaching the climax of the investigation, issued a crisp bulletin: "It is true that the miller Maillet has received and delivered good flour and that he delivered it in his own vicinity. But to compensate for this, he delivered to Pont-Saint-Esprit flour mixed with ergot of rye, after having denied that this was so. There appears to be no doubt about his responsibility."

The reaction to the news of the arrests was, of course, immediate. In Pont-Saint-Esprit there was fury. In the press there were vivid headlines announcing the apprehension of the miller and the baker, who had pawned off their unsavory wares at the expense of the unwary bakers of Pont-Saint-Esprit. LE MYSTERE DU PAIN QUI TUE EST ENFIN ELUCIDE!—THE MYSTERY OF THE MURDEROUS BREAD THAT KILLS IS AT LAST ENDED! cried one journal in flamboyant relief. Other papers, pressing in for the kill, conducted their own trials without jury and condemned and practically hoisted the two frightened men high up on the hangman's scaffold.

> The *moulin* of M. Maillet is built of old material that does not permit the proper working of the grain, and above all, treating the grain as it ought to be. Here there are no facilities for washing or cleaning. At most, it is able to grind only three hundred quintals a

month. It is for this reason it is often noted that the flour coming from this mill fails to present the same quality of fineness and whiteness that is found in that coming from more modern installations.

It is equally for this reason, without doubt, that M. Maillet furnished very little of the flour for the bakers in this vicinity.

Escorted by several impersonal *gendarmes*, the haggard and distraught men were whisked by automobile to Nîmes. M. Perrier, the regular examining magistrate, was on vacation. Substituting for him was M. Braure; the similarity of his name to that of the baker who had just been placed under arrest caused some difficulty in the public's mind as it tried to unravel the complicated threads of the story. Brought to the chambers of the substitute examining magistrate in Nîmes, in the shadow of the ruins of the Roman temples of justice and the arena where gladiators had fought to death, the men were presented with the formal charges.

"I do not contest the offenses I have committed in the *département* of Vienne," said M. Maillet, "but I don't want to make any other declarations concerning the other charges at this time."

M. Bruère confined himself to saying that he did not want to make any further declarations without the benefit of counsel.

The French system of law, knocked askew in 1789, has stumbled along for five Republics with rather shaky provision for constitutional rights. A man can be arrested without a warrant and with no knowledge of what the charges are against him. He can be held for as long as forty-eight hours without the benefit of a lawyer or anyone else being informed. The examining magistrate is a state-paid professional who designs the architecture of the case to be prosecuted without any preliminary public hearing to determine the merits of the case.

The accused can spend as much as six to nine months in prison before he is brought to formal trial. During this time the prisoner is assumed to be guilty, and the newspapers can print what they like about him, give complete details about his alleged crime, and report whatever they can find out about the police evidence.

Maillet and Bruère faced this system with bewildered acceptance. They were neither criminals nor professional con men, but frightened provincials who tried to skirt the law and found themselves facing a monstrous chain of events that culminated in what was now becoming known as the strangest case in the history of toxicology.

While they sought legal help from their jail cells, support came from other sources. The president of the distribution monopoly, the Union Meunière, in Meuse, M. Pierre Jacob, offered to stake both his sanity and his life to prove that the police and experts were wrong in finding ergot to be the cause of the tragedy. He announced that ergot is nearly always found in any flour, that it is constantly eaten in bread, and that it simply cannot be avoided. He made a flat offer to bake his own bread from rye containing the maximum possible amount of ergot, and in the presence of experts, to eat the entire loaf. "Collective madness would rage," he said, "if the experts were right and ergot were the poison."

The presidents of the Union Meunière in the *départements* of Vienne and Gard joined M. Jacob in categorically refusing to accept the theory that ergot was the cause.

One grain farmer said: "There is still a great deal of mystery to be cleared up. Through what wicked genii has *le mal des ardents*, which for two centuries has been forgotten—through what wicked genii has it reappeared? The irregularities of M. Maillet and his old and battered mill with its defective equipment are not sufficient to explain this. In every time and country there are millers without great scruples, and there are many primitive mills. How does it happen, therefore, that suddenly, in this day and age, an accident of ergotism can take place?"

Most of the victims and the villagers of Pont-Saint-Esprit felt that this was sophistry, and they were not interested. They were interested in bringing whatever culprits were involved to justice. And at last the police and the experts were coming up with something concrete. They were not permitted to forget the sword of Damocles still hanging over their heads.

The *Abbé* Jurand continued to pray, in silence, imploring Saint Saturnin, the patron of the village, to lift the "accursed bread" and its ravages from the town. Insomnia was still almost total among the victims, even those struck lightly. Some who felt they were improving lapsed back into hallucinations or convulsions, or both. There was still dread everywhere that death might strike again, and no one knew where it would be.

Many began to question just how much poison could be compressed into the bread, so that people who had eaten even small amounts had been stricken, sometimes as hard as if they had eaten generous chunks or slices. Some experts claimed that it would require twenty to fifty grams of ergot to kill a steer, fifteen to thirty to kill a horse, and five to ten grams to kill a calf. Any of these concentrations would have made the bread literally inedible.

But Commissioner Sigaud was firm in his belief that he had reached a major milestone in the case, that the responsibility could be pinned where it belonged, and that the police portion of the case, at least, could be closed. Confident also was Professor Olivier, whose further tests were revealing more presence of ergot alkaloids. In a long telephone conversation with the *juge d'instruction* he confirmed this, and felt sure that the definitive report would be ready within a few weeks.

Hardly had the call been completed, when two new events were added to the picture. First, Colonel Deniel, director of the Laboratoire Régional des Subsistance Militaires, who had been asked by the O.N.I.C. to analyze some samples of the bread, was not able to find a single trace of ergot in his analysis of the bread.

Second, Mme. Manilla Bonzi was seized with illness, convulsions, and hallucinations in the town of Saint-Julien-de-Peyrolas, close to Pont-Saint-Esprit. She was rushed in serious condition to the hospital at Nîmes. Most interesting was that she had not eaten the bread of M. Briand, but that of M. Jaussent.

NINE

THE CONSTERNATION created by the conflicting reports of the experts, disturbing as it was, did not prevent the substitute examining magistrate and Commissioner Sigaud from pressing their inquiry. For his defense M. Bruère was able to obtain the services of Maître Tessier, one of the ablest lawyers of Nîmes, whose intelligence, fairness, and wit was highly regarded by the courts in the city. He was noted for his defense of the underdog and his passion for defending the legal rights of the accused without interfering with the proper dispensation of justice. From Poitiers came Maître Grasseau, a former president of the bar in that city, to assist in the defense.

Both attorneys accompanied M. Bruère for his interrogation by the examining magistrate on September 4, 1951, when Bruère confirmed his previous statements about the *mauvaise qualité* of the grain and the general practice in the area of accepting deliveries of this sort at the end of the season. He also confirmed his rather fantastic and ephemeral method of keeping records of his grain deliveries and receipts.

Maillet, however, balked at the questioning by the examining magistrate. Although he admitted that he had signed a statement saying he had originally lied to Sigaud, he now claimed that he was forced to sign because he was physically threatened by the police, who were standing by when he was questioned at Poitiers.

The substitute examining magistrate reminded Maillet that his behavior was rather strange in contrast to his first appearance before the magistrate, when Maillet had admitted his misdemeanors and challenged only the competency of the Nîmes jurisdiction. The judge also noted that M. Maillet had made no complaint about the police tactics the day he arrived in Nîmes, whether they were those of the *police judiciaire* who helped conduct the investigation at Poitiers or those of the *gendarmes* who transported him to Nîmes. Maillet stuck fast to his revised story, saying now that he was ignorant of the fact that the local bakers in his region would not accept imperfect flour. Later, when the judge arranged a confrontation between Maillet and Bruère, Maillet insisted that he gave Bruère his own grain back in the form of flour and that he had not mixed it in with the grain of the cooperative. In several other questionings Maillet contradicted himself a considerable number of times, explaining the inconsistencies as the result of his fear of the police who questioned him. Bruère, on the other hand, admitted that he had been treated quite properly by the police. The court became convinced that the reason for Maillet's contradictions lay in the fact that it was not until he arrived in Nîmes that he became fully aware of the horror and terror of the Pont-Saint-Esprit drama and that he was desperately trying to eliminate any admissions he thought would be dangerous to him.

If Maillet panicked in this situation, it is not hard to understand why. Every headline in the French press, national and local, was after his throat; the citizenry of Pont-Saint-Esprit were in a lynching mood. Passions were running wild; indignation was boiling everywhere, from the Hôtel-Dieu to the hospitals of Nîmes, Avignon, Orange, and Montpellier, where the patients were still alternating between long hours of total rational lucidity and maniacal, violent hallucinations, and where distraught relatives sat in barren waiting rooms to hear in the distance the anguished cries of their own loved ones mixed in with the cacophony and bedlam of strangers' cries. Most painful were the visits of the parents to the children. They faced the futile and abortive task of comforting children who often did not recognize them, and who lay or thrashed about mutely on their beds, tied under the armpits with heavy canvas bands, their ankles lashed to the iron bedsteads. Others, screaming that their hands and fingers were burning up, pitifully moved their hands as if they were trying to take off pairs of gloves. One man, paying a weekly visit to his wife, found that he had to stop outside the hospital and pray for courage before he was able to enter the psychiatric ward and face the screams that greeted him.

In the hospitals, at the bedsides of the *malades*, the immensity of incertitude continued. Behind the grilled windows and iron doors in the psychiatric pavilions, the doctors continued what they themselves called *banal* treatment, simply because it was the only thing that modern medicine, anywhere in the world, could do. The fact remained that there was no specific antidote to poisoning by the ergot alkaloids, which are unstable, short-lived, difficult to identify, and in some cases still unknown in their properties. With the ergot theory now being challenged, the therapeutic possibilities were even more confused.

Dr. Pitot, always calm in the face of the inordinate confusion, tried to bring order out of chaos, fought a holding battle in the hope that some diagnostic miracle might point the way toward more specific therapy. He had been rebuilding the psychiatric section on the second floor of the hospital since 1933, until it was now a forty-bed unit in the process of recovering from World War II. During that time the Germans had removed much of his equipment which he was in the process of replacing. Even the medical supplies were still prewar. The electroencephalograph of the hospital had been appropriated by the Germans, but he was able to take some of the patients to his home, where his own EEG equipment was available. "Our feeling at the time was one of embarrassment and frustration," Dr. Pitot said some time later. "We were dealing with a situation for which we had no remedy. We had only vague references from the Middle Ages and the seventeenth century to guide us, and as we had no library at the hospital, I had to seek these out where I could."

Adding to his consternation was a new case arriving at the hospital, Mme. Bonzi, of Saint-Julien-de-Peyrolas. She reflected the classic symptoms of the *pain maudit,* but had eaten only the bread baked by M. Jaussent. She was the first patient with clearly identifiable symptoms who had not eaten the bread of M. Briand.

The laconic hospital records of the patients at Nîmes offered little guidance. They were reviewed by the doctors with a despairing sense of futility:

> E. S. 45 years. Quantity ingested: 2 kilograms of bread in 2 days. Beginning of acute condition: 18:00 hours, Aug. 26. *Hallucinations visuelles* of short duration, but repeated often. Sees a horse that comes upon him swiftly, then disappears.
>
> G. J. 40 years. Quantity ingested: 750 grams, morning and evening, August 17. Noted digestive troubles on August 19. *Hallucinations visuelles structurées:* Reports that he sees his neighbor lying in bed, being chloroformed and suffocating, that someone is in the corridor waiting to chloroform him. In addition, sees domestic animals and corpses in his room, which bring him extreme anguish. Also sees brilliant colors of great intensity.
>
> F. L. 48 years. Poisoned August 17. Quantity ingested: 300 grams. *Hallucinations visuelles structurées:* Sees many flowers, and beautiful women crowned by flowers of most vivid colors, which pass before his bed, but never respond when he speaks to them. At times, hears singing, a big choir.

Predominant were the vivid colors, flames, and huge bouquets of flowers, except when the major *crises* struck, and the scenes from Dante's *Inferno* took over the minds of the patients. Then they lay sweating and shivering, with the rancid odor of their sweat permeating the barren rooms and the hollow corridors without cease.

For Emile, the scenes were always atrocious. In his moments of calm, he knew that he was in the hôpital des fous, and as his undulating attacks came on him, he battered himself mercilessly in his attempts to escape. The staff would come on occasion to give him shock treatment, never sending less than six orderlies to hold him down. The bars on his windows still remained bent, mute testimony to the agonizing strength he had put forth in order to break away.

One day Mme. Testevin freed herself from her overwhelming task of taking care of the remaining three *malades* at La Villette, still confined to their beds, and went to the hospital at Nîmes to see Emile. She was admitted at the door of the psychiatric pavilion, locked into the waiting room with the other visitors, then ushered down the narrow corridors, past the cells where shouts, curses, and derision greeted her from both sides. Trembling, she reached the "Judas window" in Emile's room, which was totally bare except for the bed fixed securely against the wall. He was quiet, lying on his back and staring at the ceiling, giving no notice whatever of her presence. She waited patiently for some sign of recognition, but it never came. Across the hall a woman with disheveled hair was screaming. She stared at Mme. Testevin, then burst into a macabre and tuneless song. Mme. Testevin, sad and burdened, made her way back out along the corridor to return to her endless routine of scrubbing bed sheets on the hard stones of the washing well, serving tea and bouillion, and praying that somehow M. Testevin, Mme. Dezeuzes, and M. Delacquis would join Emile in some kind of miraculous recovery.

She entered through the iron gates of La Villette, now posted with a sign by Dr. Gabbai that firmly requested visitors to stay away. Even from the outside courtyard she could hear Mme. Dezeuzes still crying, and a few short cries from M. Delacquis's window as he grappled with an imaginary animal. From her husband's window she heard only silence. Twelve pairs of sheets were drying in the sun near the washing well, a sign that the Rigaud sisters were keeping up with the constant demands of the patients in her absence. With Emile in the hospital, she had been able to improve the routine somewhat, and the crises were becoming further apart now. She was even able to sleep for a few hours at a time on a cot placed at the foot of her husband's bed.

Weak as he was, M. Delacquis was experiencing long moments of rationality that were still marred, however, by the consistent compulsion to move toward the window and occasional hallucinations. But he was able to control the urge to jump out of the window, even when he was able to stop his incessant writing. His mind was turning more and more to the tragedy, since his few visitors had indicated in the briefest terms the wide extent of the event. In his mind was growing the desire to seek justice for those who had been so mercilessly stricken without warning and in such a cruel and grotesque way. When he got better, he told himself—*if* he got better—he would carry on a battle to see that all those who suffered as he did would be compensated through the leveling of responsibility where it belonged and regardless of upon whose shoulders it fell. He would commence his planning as he lay on his back, staring at the ceiling, only to find it interrupted when his comrades from the First World War joined him at his bedside, and his mind was again filled with confusion.

Down in the village M. Carle was also having more frequent moments of clarity. His compulsion to count window panes and to repeat senseless words of his own invention would die down now, sometimes for several minutes at a time. When he got better, he would think of what he could do to see that justice and compensation were brought to the victims. Neither he nor M. Delacquis knew yet the full extent of the damage throughout the town. They were assuming, on the basis of fragmentary information, that the victims numbered over a dozen; the two men were yet to learn that they could be counted by the score. Nor was M. Carle yet conscious of the frightful agony his small daughter was experiencing in Avignon. He would learn that later, when his strength grew enough for him to read the newspapers, which were kept carefully out of his reach during this time.

Mme. Charpail, mute and dissociated, remained at the table in her mother's kitchen on the rue des Quatre Coins, showing neither improvement nor decline. M. Sauvet, now fully lucid, was recalling with horror his escapade on the bridge; his wife was feeling much better, and they toasted each other with a glass of *pastis* on their deliverance.

M. Briand, in the face of a mixture of rumors, hostility, and generous support, continued his agonized appraisal of the event while his wife, who was among the more severely stricken, still lay in bed. His insomnia, along with the others, was still total and still continuing two weeks after the start of the disaster.

The base of the problem, M. Briand felt, lay in the method of control exercised by the O.N.I.C. "The controllers," he told a reporter who questioned him, "who are not always technicians, are provided by the O.N.I.C. to verify the quality of the wheat before it is threshed. This control has for its purpose to learn if the grain that is going to be put in sacks is wholesome, sound, and therefore marketable. Unfortunately, this control is so rapid, what with the utilization of combined reaping-binding machines, that there is great difficulty in seeing if there is ergot in the grain. The ergot, of course, is more often found in rye. But the flour that the bakers utilize after months of bad weather, such as we have been receiving, often contains some 2 percent bean flour and 6 to 8 percent rye flour per a one-hundred-kilo sack. We have to make the bread. We make it. There ought to exist two other inspections, one made at the storage places where the grain is placed in silos by the agricultural cooperatives, and the second at the flour mill. At this last stage the grains are anonymous, since all the different supplies are mixed together. But the miller, with the aid of testing equipment, would be able to verify the quality of the grain that he grinds. Always, it is a matter of taking a sample."

Actually, the O.N.I.C. was not as much in control of the quality of the wheat and flour as of the distribution of it, seeing that those *départements* that were deficient in grain received both flour and grain from those that had a surplus. In the cumbersome distribution system the O.N.I.C., as a government agency, and the Union Meunière, as a private monopoly, stumbled over each other in a maze of complicated legal contracts that confused more than they clarified. The result of the contract was that the Union Meunière, for profit, took over the obligation to deliver to the bakers a flour that was "*saine, loyale et marchand*," which is the French way of saying wholesome, unadulterated, and marketable. The Union was also responsible for seeing that the grain and flour conformed to legal norms. The private monopoly's duties included the general obligation of prudence and the specific obligations of seeing that the flour and the sacks in which it was transported were in good order.

A statement made by M. Arthur Geay, director of the Union Meunière of the Vienne *département*, did nothing to increase his popularity in Pont-Saint-Esprit. He told the police investigators, "I am officially ignorant if there has been any fraud concerning the quality of the merchandise delivered by M. Maillet. . . ." If the president of the monopoly in the area where the grain came from was "officially ignorant," it was asked, *why* was he ignorant, and what were his job and his responsibilities?

There was a vague feeling along Grande Rue and the Boulevard Gambetta that the investigation was not proceeding as it should, that someone or something was being protected or covered up, and that political excuses were replacing honest and vigorous inquiry. If strings were being pulled, there was no real evidence of it. The toxicologists were working with all the energy at their command. The *juge d'instruction*, the *commissaire*, the *police judiciaire*, the mobile brigades, and the *gendarmerie* were spading up every possible clue they could uncover. The doctors in the hospitals were using every weapon, feeble as it might be, at their disposal, and the local doctors in the village were still mainly sleepless and on the verge of breakdowns themselves. The fact was that everybody concerned, including M. Briand and the victims themselves, was still fighting one of the most elusive phantoms in medical history, the battle inevitably leading to frustrations, recriminations, and the directing of gunfire against their own troops.

Dr. Gabbai, his dossier of notes growing bigger by the day, took time off to drive to Nîmes to meet his wife and family on their return from the Pyrenees by train. Although the sporadic outbreaks were still occurring days after the nightmarish night of *l'éclosion brutale*, the interns from Nîmes, Montpellier, and Avignon were making it possible for him, Dr. Vieu, and Dr. Channac to get some relief from the pressures, even in the face of the continuing chaos. The maximum each doctor could handle was an average of four patients an hour, and all the local doctors had been handling approximately eighty patients a day. For the drive to Nîmes, about an hour away, Dr. Gabbai took some amphetamine for the first time since the disaster began. Driving this distance, he was afraid of falling asleep at the wheel, after nine days without going to bed. It was the first and only time he took medication himself, until on the twelfth day without sleep, the burden of the massive job he and the other doctors were faced with struck him with an unexpectedly vicious impact. Suddenly and without warning he was felled by a cerebral spasm and a condition of the blood vessels known as hemiplegia, which is a paralysis of one side of the body. He was flattened for two days, during which time he continued his efforts to solve the mystery, collating his notes and charts, conferring with Dr. Giraud and Dr. Latour from Montpellier, who were relentlessly studying the cases in the hope of clarifying the enigma.

Both men from Montpellier were urbane, distinguished, aristocratic. They stood out in sharp contrast in the provincial town, as they made their way through the crooked streets, and up and down the dark, twisted, stone stairs of the villagers' homes. They would return at times to their studies in Montpellier to assess and evaluate the data they had collected, Dr. Latour would shut himself in his elegant, tasteful apartment on the Boulevard du Jeu de Paume; Dr. Giraud in his inviting house on the Enclos Tissié in the academic cloister of the ancient and venerable University of Montpellier. Late in the night the men would study the notes they had collected. Dr. Latour worked at a handsome antique desk, a dim light reflecting in the impeccable parquet floors. Around him were ancient Roman curios, and after his long hours he would sip a glass of port and try to bring sense to an imponderable mystery. Dr. Giraud, several years his senior, worked in a more cluttered study, surrounded by books of literature, theater, and medicine. He was a precise and thorough man, with a passion for detail and accuracy augmenting his broad literary and scientific interests.

Both doctors worked in an atmosphere of distinguished medical and academic tradition. Not only had spice merchants of ancient days brought back to Montpellier medicines and herbs from the Orient, but the works of Hippocrates had been translated, and a center for medical learning had been created there even before the University of Montpellier had begun. The center became one of the first medical schools in the world. At the university, Rabelais had concluded his medical studies in 1538. But all the tradition, the knowledge, and the intelligence concentrated there could do little for the victims of Pont-Saint-Esprit—nor could any other medical center do anything further under the conditions existing at the time. Both men would, however, with the assistance of the doctors and interns working in the field, continue their efforts to define the plague in all its complexities and subtleties for the French Academy of Medicine.

The most distressing fact for everybody concerned was the inefficacy of medicines. Whenever sleep would come to a patient, there would be some improvement, but sleep itself was the one impossibility in the face of the almost total insomnia. All sedation continued to be ineffective. At the hospitals the more severe therapy of electro-shock treatments and ACTH (adrenocorticotrophic hormone) brought absolutely no relief.

The two doctors dug more deeply into the mysteries of ergot, scraping up every piece of information on modern research of the drug as well as on historical ergotism. Ergot, under control, had many useful purposes. Ergot running wild was disaster. In examining the fast-growing data, they found the absence of many signs that would indicate other drugs as the source of the poisoning. Mercury fungicides had been suggested, but there was no kidney damage or ashen color to the mouth so typical of mercury poisoning; nor were there the sore gums, the loosening of teeth, and the strong metallic taste that accompanied it. In mercury-poisoning victims death was inevitably caused by the toxic action on the kidney, the site of the highest concentration of the mineral. These renal lesions were consistently obvious and manifold. Here, there was no such evidence.

In narcotic poisoning there was frequently evidence of paralysis, and many narcotics brought about strong erotic syndromes which were totally absent in the Pont-Saint-Esprit cases.

New pharmaceutical studies of ergot had revealed the multiplicity, the diversity, and the variety of the chemical composition of the substance. The natural form of the drug had shown a surprisingly active capacity to engender new and undiscovered properties; its instability made it so elusive that toxicologists were never sure with what they were working. The alkaloids of ergot were capable of disappearing with alarming rapidity. They were numerous, and not all their properties were known. The natural forms were more powerful than the synthetic. Laboratory tests had shown that not more than 5 percent of an intravenous dose could be accounted for in the body, even five minutes after an injection.

The clinical aspects of historical ergotism were diverse, and the Pont-Saint-Esprit syndromes continued to match strikingly with the forms noted in previous centuries, whether convulsive or gangrenous, paresthetic or hallucinatory, simple or mixed.

Reading a description of the ergot epidemic of Marbourg in 1595, both Giraud and Latour noticed the striking similarities.

> The sickness habitually begins with a tingling and prickling of the skin, then the fingers and toes contract or expand with a strong rigidity. . . . During the crises, there are sensations of intense burning and freezing cold. . . .
>
> The intellectual troubles are very varied . . . hallucinations which render the sick very dangerous and make it necessary to close them in or tie them up . . . there is profuse sweating.

One medical analyst, writing in 1874, summed up the perplexities facing Dr. Giraud and Dr. Latour with his own puzzlement:

> We are obliged to declare that we do not yet have sufficient knowledge of the nature of this toxic agent, and to admit that, following the conditions of time and place, the poison is able to vary not only in its force and energy, but in its pathogenic modes, under the influence, without doubt, of its association of diverse other causes of alternation among the grains and flour, whether parasitic in nature or not.

Thus, in 1951, the doctors continued to face the same enigma as in 1874—or in the Middle Ages, or in the beginning of history.

Chafing under his enforced rest in bed, and experiencing difficulty in speaking because of his attack—a condition which was to stay with him for many years—Dr. Gabbai broke down his notes in careful, documented order. In addition to the charts for each patient, classified according to the intensity of the case, Dr. Gabbai chronicled his observations over the long sleepless hours on the streets and in the houses of the *malades*. He wrote:

> Absorption took place during a single day. The bread certainly contained a high proportion of poison, for the amounts eaten were often very small. In this first phase, the symptoms were generalized . . . after some hours the symptoms become more clearly defined, and most of the patients presented digestive disturbances, along with a depressive state, with anguish and slight agitation. Particularly noted was the state of nausea, with diffuse abdominal pain; less often noted were vomiting and diarrhea. There was often a sensation of distressing pharyngeal constriction.
>
> Disturbance of the autonomic nervous system accompanied the digestive disorders—hot flashes, followed by the impression of

"cold waves," with periods of intense sweating . . . the patients were pale and often showed a regular bradycardia (40 to 50 beats a minute). Temperature of most patients low, both in morning and evening (97.8–98.2). Arterial tension in general rather low. . . . Sometimes disquieting fall in blood pressure during fainting attacks. . . . Mydriasis very frequent . . . diminution of the light reflex.

Several complaints of pain at nape of the neck, more rarely true headaches. Insomnia—constant. Diffuse, subhepatic abdominal pain, burning sensations throughout the whole of the digestive tract. Patients pale, limp, inconspicuous trembling of the extremities. Many recover with only these symptoms. Others, worse after a 48-hour lull. Sharp tingling, pallor, and cold in the extremities . . . painful paresthesia and cramps in the calves. Some had severe fainting attacks with imperceptible pulse . . . low and feeble arterial tension. Logorrhea, psychomotor agitation, and absolute insomnia nearly always presaged the appearance of mental disorders. Themes of hallucinations included visuals of animals and flames . . . many cases followed by dreamy delirium. Delirium seemed to be systematized, with animal hallucinations and self-accusation, sometimes mystical and macabre.

Every attempt at restraint increased the agitation. Some muscular spasms, recalling those of tetanus. . . . During this stage, abundant sweating. Duration of periods of delirium, varied . . . those who died did so of cardiovascular collapse and muscular spasm. Gangrene noted . . . some women with hemorrhages . . . some with premature menstruation . . .

The hemorrhages were a new symptom, but they fell into place among the symptoms of historical ergotism as surely as pieces in a picture puzzle. At Pont-Saint-Esprit three-quarters of the women victims encountered this trouble.

On the heels of this new development came a flood of skin eruptions, and again the symptoms continued to affirm the close similarity of the disease to historical ergotism. The skin eruptions, appearing late in the progress of the disease, were bothersome but not serious. Their duration, however, was to be extended over a long period of time.

The eruptions experienced by the patients who had eaten the bread had their roots in a series of circumstances which began to come to the forefront as the new symptom appeared.

When M. Briand had begun to sort out the samples of *le pain maudit* to prepare to send them to the police laboratory for analysis, he noticed that he felt a burning sensation on the tips of his fingers. Later, when he touched his hands to his face, the burning sensation happened again, more severely. He noticed Dr. Channac's car in front of his shop, and immediately called him in and told him about it. Dr. Channac made a note of the incident and returned to his office. Later that evening, Dr. Channac returned to M. Briand's bakery and told him that he felt the same kind of sensation on his own fingers and face after handling the bread. The bread was labeled and sent on to the laboratory in Marseilles. The eczema created by the contact continued over many weeks.

Beyond that, several persons taking care of the sick reported that they suffered from a burning sensation and eczema after touching the patients. Mayor Hebrard, after his long series of visits to the sick both in Pont-Saint-Esprit and in the hospitals, noted a strong sensation of burning on his hands after shaking hands with many of the patients.

Georges Gillot, the investigator for the Department of Health, noticed that he broke out in a rash during his confiscation of the samples of flour from the supplies of M. Bousquet in Bagnols-sur-Cèze. Corroborating this, another inspector from the Department of Health encountered the same symptoms after he had handled the samples of flour coming from M. Griotti, the baker whose bread had been the forerunner to the Pont-Saint-Esprit disaster.

M. Gillot then used his own arms as a testing laboratory, trying out the different samples of M. Griotti's flour on his skin. Over a period of several weeks he rubbed the labeled and coded samples on his skin, charting whether the sample created an eczema condition or not. He concluded from the results that at least two sacks under seal with M. Griotti were still toxic many weeks after the original flurry of illnesses connected with his bread.

But none of this helped to solve the new question mark brought on by the conflicting reports from Dr. Ollivier's laboratory and the military laboratory under Colonel Deniel. Ollivier took a firm stand against the statement issued by the colonel, insisting that traces of ergot had been found both in the viscera and in the bread samples he had examined. He also commented wryly on the brash offer by M. Jacob, the Union Meunière executive who had offered to eat bread especially baked with ergot. "I'm afraid I'd have another autopsy on my hands," was Ollivier's remark when he learned of M. Jacob's statement.

Just when it appeared that a giant battle was looming up between the two laboratories, the colonel and the professor quickly settled their differences. They issued a joint statement that did nothing to advance the unraveling of the mystery, but which at least removed another roadblock in the way of keeping momentum going in the investigation.

> Only the Laboratoire Interrégional de Police Scientifique de Marseilles has been authorized by the judiciary police to make an analysis concerning the affair of Pont-Saint-Esprit. It is the only laboratory to have received all the elements necessary to continue the investigation, the only one to receive the samples placed officially under seal: bread, flour, viscera, reports from the clinic, and autopsies.
>
> On the request of the O.N.I.C. the military laboratory at Marseilles has analyzed only one portion of one sample of bread, which has not been held under official judiciary seal, and this single analysis does not provide enough information to reach a general conclusion concerning this affair.
>
> The directors of both laboratories concerned, whose signatures appear below, after a complete exchange of points of view, and in perfect accord, submit this joint communiqué to dispel the confusion that could arise from certain unfounded interpretations which are insufficiently clarified.

Thus ended one of the first battles among the experts, but others were already being formed. As each new controversy was made public, another merciless wave of confusion would spread among the townspeople, already staggering from a burden they or anyone else would hardly be equipped to bear.

In the village the only topic of conversation continued to be *le pain maudit*. Fantastic accusations flooded the cafés. Dozens of hypotheses were advanced; few had any relation to reality. Yet what was real in a disaster which was as mysterious to the experts as it was to the layman? The villagers had read so many news reports, heard so many rumors, listened to so many tales that they were dismally despairing of finding an answer. The reality they knew was reflected in the huge pennant strung across the ancient portals of the Hôtel-Dieu, which in large black letters named the doctors and the pharmacy assigned each day to *les services de nuit,* or through the reprises of the cries, the tears, the maledictions, the trembling, the delirium, and the clamor that continued to show itself sporadically in the streets.

They were beginning to be released from the hospitals now, a few at a time. They were welcomed back with love and affection, but not unalloyed. Underneath the affection was a layer of fear, the inescapable thought that a relapse might come at any minute; that the awful scenes of the night of the Apocalypse might return again.

The fear was not unjustified. Mme. Isabelle Payan, returning to her husband and small children on the Grande Rue was filled with joy after the long days and nights in a strait jacket in the hospital at Nîmes. Her progress was good. Sleep was returning to her. Her mind was still filled with the unbearable sounds of the psychiatric wing, but the memory was fading in the warmth and security of her home.

Their apartment in the old village was modest. M. Payan had just recently moved his family from the Vaucluse, having found a job on the Donzère-Mondragon project.

The first recurrence was short-lived. Mme. Payan ran to the window without warning, flung it open, and came to her senses just at the moment she started to jump. She could not explain where the impulse came from and shuddered at the thought of what would have happened if she had followed it. A few moments later she found herself suddenly going to the wardrobe, opening the door, and trying to enter it.

"Isabelle, what are you doing?" said her husband.

"Excuse me," she said. "I thought it was time to take the train!"

By Saturday she felt better. The incredible azure-blue of the Midi sky, the crisp, fresh October air, and the release from the anguish of the hospital all combined to revivify her spirits and bring her refreshed hope. The market sprawled along the center strip of the Boulevard Gambetta was the same as she had remembered it: the trinkets, the mountains of greens, the shoes, the clothes, the hardware, the pots and pans, the pottery, the crowded paths between the stalls, the noise, the confusion. All that was lacking was the usual gaiety. No one in the village could forget so soon; no one could be expected to do so.

She gained courage and confidence among the familiar sights and sounds. She approached a fruit and vegetable stall, where mounds of local grapes were displayed. She bought a kilo and placed them in her shopping bag.

It happened so suddenly that no one, including Mme. Payan was aware of how it happened. With a scream, she threw her shopping sack to the ground, tore off her hat, and flung her arms wildly about her.

"Stand back! Don't touch me! Let me alone!" she yelled. "You want to kill me, to poison me! I know it! Assassins!"

Then, as suddenly as it had come on, the attack subsided. It was not the last time that she would relapse into the darkness she thought she had left forever. "I feel that I would like to die!" she later said.

René Argellier, too, exchanged the cruel, tight bindings of the strait jacket for the warmth of his home when it was thought that he was cured. A smallish man of thirty-six years, with a pale, drawn visage, he returned hopefully from the echoing hallways of the hospital at Nîmes to his family farm on the road to the Ardeche. Speaking to a sympathetic reporter, he told the story in his own words:

> Monsieur, *je suis un homme fini.*
>
> I remained a month at the *maison des fous* at Nîmes. They felt I was cured. Last Thursday, after having eaten my dinner, I realized I had no more cigarettes. I got on my bicycle to go to the *tabac* to get some. But at the doorway of the shop the sickness overcame me again. I saw the house tumble down on top of me. The stones and the timbers were crushing my body. The people standing by ran over to me and held me down. My hallucinations continued. Bombs were exploding all around me, and little goblins were attacking me with blood-red needles like pikes, stabbing me all over. The men rushed me to the Hôtel-Dieu, where I spent the night tied to the bed. But in the morning I had become very calm again.
>
> The only difference between this crisis and the preceding one is that I recognized the people who surrounded me and sought to take care of me.

He recalled his first attack, when he felt as if he had been placed on a pyre and saw train after train approaching him, then receding, and then a truck which pursued him on the bridge at Pont-Saint-Esprit, flinging him into the river.

> There is no doubt that these hours of senseless nightmares profoundly disturbed me. But I believe I suffered more when morning came, with my mind clear, my body calm, and I found myself in a narrow white cell with the thick bars in front of me, tied by leather straps to an iron bed. I would cry out that I was better, that I was well, but they would pass by my door without looking or coming back for me.
>
> The doctors have told me that I must be patient—that it will perhaps be five years before I recover my equilibrium. I will never be able to wait that long.

The toast that M. Sauvet and his wife made to each other in *pastis* was ill-timed. A few days afterward, the genial and well-liked *garagiste* rose in the night and pedaled off on his bicycle as Mme. Sauvet roused her neighbors to give chase in a car. They found him hours later, confused and apologetic, deeply mournful about the worry he had caused.

There were other incidents, too, enough to fray the nerves of everyone in the village, who had been now for more than three weeks without respite from continued shock. There was the man at the market who suddenly greeted an old friend by stopping him next to the Fontaine de la Navigation to say: "Look at my feet—do you hear the pretty music coming from them? Isn't it strange? And see the beautiful antennae there?"

There was the thirteen-year old who without warning began breaking up the furniture in his home. Or the mother and son whose cases had been extremely light, and who were suddenly rushed to the hospital at Nîmes.

There were the scores of villagers who were not sick, had no hallucinations, experienced no *idée fixe,* felt no pain, but lay on their beds each night for over twenty nights, their eyes wide open, their thoughts churning, their dread and apprehension rising—and no sleep whatever. The sheer agony of the total insomnia was almost unbearable; the smarting eyes, the aching muscles, the agonizing void of total wakefulness was as tortuous as for those who remained in or were returned to the cells in the psychiatric pavilions. Conscious all the time of the voluminous news of the affair of "the accursed bread," the half-sick *malades* tossed and twisted in their beds with the unblockable fear and apprehension of what was going to happen next.

The brief battle of the experts and the truce that followed was simply another stinging rebuff to impose further uncertainty on their exhausted minds. Professor Ollivier's follow-up letter to the *juge d'instruction* was of no comfort either, even though it did bring an air of finality to the entire mystery:

Ministère de l'Interieur Laboratoire Interrégional de Police Scientifique de MARSEILLES	Le Directeur du Laboratoire Interrégional de Police Scientifique de Marseilles à M. PERRIER juge d'instruction Tribunal de 1° instance; Palais de Justice NÎMES

Object: a/s Aff. de Pont-St-Esprit
Reference: Ar. Chron N° Chro 2445
Monsieur le Juge,
Following our telegram of the Thirtieth of August, 1951, and in execution of your ordinances concerning the affair of Pont-St-Esprit, we have the honor to bring to your attention the new results, actually bringing together the deductions from the series of chemical, biological and microscopic examinations relative to the analysis of 22 different specimens (bread, viscera, etc.) and representing an actual total of some 100 groups of tests.

These new examinations bring confirmation of the presence of a substance possessing the toxicological characteristics of the active principles of ergot, parasite of cereals in the following samples:

1° VISCERA
MISON-RIEU Dog
2° BREAD SAMPLES
Jaussent-August 12
Mison-August 16
Moulin-August 16
Moulin-August 18
Briand-August 20

The report went on to disclose, however, that the other specimens among the twenty-two samples were negative as far as the presence of ergot was concerned. Was the elusive chemical disintegration, for which ergot was known, so volatile that it had already escaped from the samples by the time the laboratory was able to test them? This was a major point that would have to be examined in great detail. For the moment, however, the letter concluded:

> These results are still awaiting further tests, and do not permit fully satisfactory conclusions by themselves, notably needing the confrontation of the interpretations revealed by the application of different methods and techniques, thus making a series of complementary experiments necessary.
>
> The definitive report will be sent to you with the minimum of delay at the completion of our new experiments.
>
> Marseilles, October 15, 1951
> (Signed) Dr. Ollivier

Regardless of the tentative tone of the letter, regardless of the mysterious qualities of ergot, and regardless of its capacity to resist medical therapy, the threat had been smoked out and recognized, and the enemy was engaged—even if only with toy guns and tin armor as protection. There was no real satisfaction when the news of this letter was released, but a bizarre form of stability was established for the first time since the day of disaster had arrived. This pseudostability, however, could not possibly protect the *Spiritpontains* from the formidable shoals surrounding them. Two violent gusts of wind set their unseaworthy craft reeling out to sea again.

The first gust came with the news that Joseph Portal, a fellow-townsman of long standing, had died in the Hôpital Psychiatrique de Mondevergues, the fifth fatality of *le pain maudit*, and so certified by his attending physician.

The second gust was accompanied by front-page headlines in practically every newspaper in France. A hydraulic engineer, who was technical counsel to nearly four hundred French villages on the problems of water supply, engineer-counsel of the Ministry of Justice, and consultant to the French and American military services on the establishment of water supply, released a blunt and shocking report that said without evasion or equivocation: The water supply of Pont-Saint-Esprit, and the water supply *alone,* is the cause of the five deaths, the victims rendered insane, and the other sickness raging through the little village on the Rhône.

TEN

THE HYDRAULIC engineer's name was M. Louis-Claude Vincent. His report was written with passionate indignation, oddly out of tune with what might be expected from an engineering mind. He took great pains to see that his theory was outlined and sent to an impressive list of authorities, including public officials, judges, politicians, and newspapers. He underlined with almost frantic emphasis that the water was the exclusive cause of the poisonings, beyond any doubt. He went further than that. He indicated that the water would *continue* to ravage the populations because of its toxicity. It contained, he claimed, important quantities of arsenic and nitrites. He did not explain just how the arsenic might so mysteriously appear. He stated that the source of the supply was a public scandal, and that he hoped "in the interest of the martyred population that the truth will finally triumph."

Bursting into a peak of elegance, he said that "as in the time of the *Bas Empire*, and in the image of the doctors of the Byzance who philosophized on the sexes of the angels as the Turks climbed their ramparts, our modern doctors prefer to offer dissertations on an imponderable ergotism, ignoring at present the poisonous ammoniacs which continue their work of creating *de folie* and *de mort*."

If there were anything designed to pulverize the last remaining semblance of calm, this statement was it. Sales of wine sky-rocketed throughout the region; housewives cooked in nothing but wine, or even *pastis*. In the cafés, this favorite beverage of the Provençal was served straight and syrupy, clinging to the roof of the mouth, but infinitely safer than in its customary state, mixed with water. Even the journalists, collected daily at the Café de la Bourse, shuddered at the thought of eating anything that was mixed with water.

Up until now they had their jokes and deceits that continued to serrate the nerves of the populace. One reporter brought a girl in from Avignon, dressed her as a nurse, placed her sister in a bed in his hotel room to simulate a scene of bedside agony for his press photographer. Another created a fake funeral to get a picture to return to his paper. Still another returning on a furlough to Paris, as he phrased it, painted the words PONT ST. ESPRIT on a sweat shirt, and staggered into his office with a loaf of bread under his arm.

On the release of the information from M. Vincent, the press corps became muffled and subdued. The assignment to Pont-Saint-Esprit lost its glamor.

M. Vincent built his case with extreme attention to unimportant detail and irrelevant fact. Even the national minister of health was impressed. The engineer had been charged by a group of industrial planners to study the possibilities for a new pharmaceutical plant, to be established in the region, and testing the water of Pont-Saint-Esprit was part of his assignment.

"On the Twenty-fourth of September, I presented myself at the town hall of the village to obtain the preliminary information on the water of Pont-Saint-Esprit," M. Vincent said. "There I learned that the bacteriological analysis of the water was satisfactory, but that no chemical analysis had been made since 1946. But the analysis at that time showed evidence that the water was already charged with chlorine and sulphuric acid. These preliminary confirmations made, I went to visit the water installation and perceived with astonishment that it was next to the gas works."

He went on to explain that a subterranean gallery of the gas works was some twenty meters below the ground, passing within a few meters of the water supply. Through a faulty mechanism, which M. Vincent went to great lengths to explain, the debris from the gas manufacturing unit could have brought arsenic and nitrites to the water supply. "This is what has provoked the catastrophe," he said firmly, with still no explanation of why arsenic should be present.

After the immediate and violently apprehensive reaction to his theory had subsided, the questions began to come. Aside from Mme. Bonzi and one other family, all sickness seemed to be established as coming from the bread of M. Briand. Why, then, was not the entire town poisoned? Further, why did the symptoms, overall, reflect only the symptoms of classic historical ergotism? Beyond that, no trace whatever of arsenic or nitrites had been found, to say nothing of the lack of correspondence between the symptoms demonstrated by the sick and those resulting from arsenic or nitrite poisoning. Arsenic, especially, was easy and clear to trace in the system. Why, also, was the mass outbreak sudden and traumatic, rather than a long sickness of attrition, if the water were at fault? There was no evidence whatever of a slow and insidious poisoning.

Further, a report from M. Bataillon, *médecin-directeur de la Santé du Gard* proved conclusively that the water supply had been regularly surveyed from the chemical as well as the bacteriological point of view. The results were clearly acceptable:

> Sample of July 25, 1951: A la borne fontaine de
> La Marie: EAU POTABLE
> Sample of October 1, 1951: A la borne fontaine
> de la Place: EAU POTABLE

Other analyses indicated that the color, odor, deposits, and mineral and vegetable content were fully compatible with normal standards, and there was no reason to have concern over the water supply. After the authorities confirmed and reconfirmed these conclusions, M. Vincent's intense but brief limelight was dimmed as quickly as it had flooded the atmosphere, and no more was heard of the theory.

Although the possibility of an entirely different source of the poisoning from the bread bolstered M. Maillet's and M. Bruère's cases, it did nothing but stiffen Commissioner Sigaud's resolve to support the ergot theory, and to prosecute Maillet and Bruère to the full extent of the law. By now the lawyers of the miller and the baker from the north were pleading eloquently, and not without reason, for their clients to be *mis en liberté provisoire*, the French equivalent of being released on bail. There was not sufficient evidence, they argued cogently. The two men were being held in jail on extremely thin pretenses. Thin as it was, the shadow of doubt cast by the hydraulic engineer spurred hopes of the men gaining their freedom, further supported by a long communiqué issued by L'Association de la Meunière Français.

In it, the millers' organization insisted that the presence of ergot was not formally proven by the experts, and that the properties of the drug when it was employed pharmaceutically made it evident that no one could have eaten the bread under any circumstances.

Ergot would only be toxic, the communiqué went on to say, in doses of four to ten grams. Bread containing that much of a dosage of ergot, according to the millers, would have presented such characteristics as an extremely nauseous odor, a repellent taste, and a dark gray color which would have been immediately obvious. But the bread had been, without any doubt whatever, highly savory, and no person who ate it had shown any real indication of not wanting to do so.

"The responsibility of the miller," the communiqué continued, "is therefore not established in any formal way. In the absence of such proof, there remain only two hypotheses: (1) an accident after the flour was placed in the sack, when it was poisoned in transport, a hypothesis difficult to maintain because the flour was sealed at the mill; and (2) an act of a criminal—*the theory that remains the most plausible*."

Since the villagers had barely recovered from the shocking accusation of the water supply, they were left reeling and shocked again by this energetic resurrection of the criminal theory. Any theory that allowed for the strong possibility of the rampage to continue, painfully increased the tensions on the nerves of the townspeople, which were now stretched tighter than a fine piano wire.

Meanwhile, further investigation of the mill of M. Maillet

failed to uncover any great irregularities, either fraudulent bookkeeping or incompetent milling of the grain. In fact, one investigator in his official report commented:

"M. Maillet is a well-regarded miller without any great dynamism in his character, who never draws particular attention to himself. One would not generally classify him as a *fraudeur*. A sample of flour taken from him in January, 1950, did not lead to any particular observation in the laboratory.

"M. Bruère also is considered as a *boulanger serieux*, and he has no record of previous infractions."

The investigator added that Maillet's mill was considered one of the better in the *département*, in the opinion of other professionals, who indicated that there was *always* the presence of ergot in feeble quantities in any grain, but that it was harmless.

In contrast to this benign report, the official appraisal of the cooperative of Saint-Julien-l'Ars, with which neither of the men held in jail had any connection, was rather startling: "We have confirmed in this establishment on a shelf in the hall of the first floor three packets of arsenic, sealed, and twelve packets of the toxic hexachlorocyclohexane. The wrapping of these packets was in a bad state, and would permit the toxic powder to pour out on the sacks destined to carry the grain. In another part of the same hallway, the sacks destined to carry the grain were sitting on bags of chemical fertilizer and bottles of Gésarol [dichloro-diphenyl-trichloro-ethane, the technical name for DDT]."

With this report, were graphic photographs of the conditions in the cooperative.

Seizing on this and other evidence, the barristers representing Maillet and Bruère pressed their appeal for the release, at least on a provisional basis, for the two men. M. Tessier, always eloquent and persuasive, presented his plea in the form of a letter:

> In the name of Monsieur le Batonnier Grasseau, and in mine, I have the honor of asking you to place *en liberté provisoire* M. BRUÈRE. . . .
>
> The dolorous affair of the poisonings of Pont-Saint-Esprit has provoked all the region and even the entire country. . . .
>
> But if the incriminated ought to be actively investigated—if they are truly culpable—they should not be permitted to remain in de-

> tention when the responsibility is not actually determined, and when they have been seized too quickly and without proof. . . .
>
> In effect: (1) Contrary to the writings of the *Commissaire de Police Judiciaire,* nothing has established that the cause of the poisoning is *ergot de seigle.* Professor Ollivier, in his communication of August 30, 1951, has not said that. The report of Colonel Deniel, chief of the Laboratoire Régional des Subsistances Militaires has clearly said that ergot was not able to be placed in evidence. . . .
>
> Let us say again that in their minds, the experts, their conviction not firm, do not hesitate to envisage a long series of diverse hypotheses, requiring further research of extremely long duration . . . At length, it is necessary to *demonstrate,* and this has not been done, that the ergot, if it is present, *is in sufficient quantity to be toxic.* (2) Further, even if the ergot is able to be incriminated—and the dossier proves nothing, absolutely nothing to establish this—it would be necessary to prove not only that the toxic bread originated in Maillet's flour, but that this flour came from the grain delivered by Bruère.
>
> Nothing permits us to think this.
>
> The dossier in this regard is empty of proof.
>
> It carries with it a collection of imprecise declarations, and discordant contradictions which fail to establish in any certain fashion the origin of the flour employed.

The letter continued, pointing out that the evidence was not only incomplete, but conflicting, and that the men would certainly remain at their homes and be available at any time when the judge needed them for further inquiry.

But the *juge d'instruction* remained firm, in spite of the fact that the arguments were not only persuasive but in some cases incontrovertible. Further, the public pressure to pin down the responsibility packed far more steam than the sympathy for the two men who had admitted some indiscretions, even if without intent to damage. Intent or not, the results were so sweeping and tragic that the effect dwarfed any cause that might be uncovered. The decision of the judge, hanging on the balance of fragmentary expertise, was agonizing in either direction. It demanded the wisdom of Solomon, the compassion of a saint, the firmness of a field commander.

Professor Ollivier, in the meanwhile, had added two new experts to bolster his reasearch, to the relief of the police, who were champing with further impatience in the face of pressures from all sides. Professor Dumazert, professor of chemistry at the University of Marseilles, and Professor Pelissier, professor of botany at the same institution, joined him as the investigation continued. They were to be joined later by the noted toxicologist M. Kohn-Abrest, a former director of the toxicological laboratory of the Préfecture de Police de la Seine and an expert in the service of the Tribunal in Paris. It was an impressive group, and their first statement as a team was that "the affair of the poisonings of Pont-Saint-Esprit was without precedent in the annals of toxicology." Most experts around the world agreed with that. From other countries came other advice and suggestions. An Italian doctor insisted it was hashish, planted in great quantity by a criminal. A British doctor was sure it was poison arising from chemicals added to the flour for the purpose of bleaching it. Both these suggestions were able to be definitively ruled out later.

Another expert, of an entirely different genre, was the Marquis de Saint-Génies, whose name was well known in the nearby, mysterious plains of the Camargue, where legends, Gypsies, and French cowboys blend in with the atmosphere of magic that surrounds the countryside. As supreme delegate to l'Ordre Kabbalistique de la Rose-Croix, this mystic's advice was sought on every matter from weddings to reincarnation, and he was generous with his advice. He was a great admirer of George Sand, who liked to dress as a man. He, in turn, complemented the habits of the famous author by dressing like a woman. His position was that no forces of malediction were responsible for the tragedy of Pont-Saint-Esprit, even if the plague did appear to be resurrected from the Middle Ages. He sharply rapped the knuckles of one *Spiritpontain* who tried to blame the entire matter on witchcraft and sorcery.

"Pont-Saint-Esprit is not an area predisposed to magic," he said, "even though the village has been plunged *en plein moyen âge*, and has been struck by the wind of the devil. It is a tragic accident." The marquis' words carried much weight. He was one of the few members of the occult profession who refused to accept a fee or a contribution.

All through the time that the battle lines among the theorists, police and scientists, were being formed, most of the victims who had survived were showing a slow improvement. At first it was almost imperceptible, since the promising signs were pushed into the background by the more dramatic and violent setbacks that punctuated the scenes. But hope slowly began to rise along Grande Rue, in the church, the cafés, and the market place.

The day came—while Professor Ollivier was preparing his temporary reports, while Commissioner Sigaud was pressing the inquiry against Maillet and Bruère, while the theorists from outside the region were advancing their long-distance suggestions—the day came when Mme. Testevin could sleep for hours at a time, when Mme. Dezeuzes could stop crying and close her eyes, when M. Testevin could forget the fantasies of his feasts and the sounds of the imaginary chase and hunt, to nourish himself with long draughts of sleep. The necessity for steeping the dried lime flowers for tea became less frequent, and La Villette even had brief moments of cheer as the convalescence began. M. Delacquis was able to straighten his fingers, stiff from incessant writing, and look at the window without the agony of trying to resist the impulse to jump. The hallucinations were gone now, and sheer exhaustion and weakness replaced them. All the members of La Villette were ashen and drawn, but their appetites began to increase, the anguish of their minds began to diminish, and above all, the capacity to sleep returned, which created an almost excruciating bliss. Even Emile, though pale and thin as a ghost, toothless all along the forefront of his mouth, and ravaged by the convulsions that had accompanied his terrifying hallucinations, was able to sleep in a hospital room without bars, and to begin to eat.

Tiny Marie-Joseph Carle returned to her home; she was now scrawny and pathetic. But she rebounded quickly, with the resilience of children. M. Carle, after twenty-one days of sleeplessness, had at long last conquered his compulsion to count and to mutter senseless words. He read the newspapers his wife had kept for him, and his indignation rose faster than his physical strength returned.

At the Moulin farm, Mme. Moulin no longer saw the frightening *tête du mort,* and M. Moulin, weak from his days in the hospital, was able to sit up now as well as sleep. The father and mother of young Joseph, crushed by the death of their son and hopeless in their anguish, bitterly resolved that they would try to find the origin of the tragedy so that others would not suffer as they had.

The vines at both the Moulin and Testevin vineyards were bursting with grapes at harvest time, and neighbors rushed in to help, while the convalescent proprietors weakly gave directions from their beds.

No one knows exactly who first conceived of the idea, but several different plans for organizing an association of the victims seemed to be spontaneously amalgamated. The association would try to bring about justice in the case and attempt to indemnify the legitimate victims, whose loss of time, of money, of crops, of services, of life, and of limb was so staggering that it would be impossible to assess it accurately; the conscious pain and suffering could never be measured in terms of money. The founders of the association wanted justice first, and only then would they attempt to obtain some sort of indemnification for the bulk of the poor among them who had become hopelessly in debt, the farmers who had lost their crops, the proprietors whose vineyards had suffered damage, the laborers who had been unable to work, the widows who would have to struggle on alone, and the shopkeepers who had been forced to close their stores.

For the most part, the illnesses began to subside after the twenty-first day, except for the most seriously ill and those who suffered severe relapses. With convalescence came the outbreaks of eczema, the hemorrhages of the women, and the cyclical return of dizziness and hallucinations. Not all were so lucky; many remaining barely functional in the face of their physical or psychological damage, would retain their scars the rest of their lives.

Mayor Hebrard seized on the idea for an association of victims and fostered it. Emerging as the two most motivated and energetic men in the articulation of the idea were M. Carle and M. Delacquis. They were intelligent, strong-willed, and tenacious men, who could organize, direct, and still work tirelessly in their own occupations, who had the respect of the community, and whose background and experience were broad and nonprovincial. They were physically weak, almost hopelessly so. But each was convinced that only in unity was there a chance for indemnification and a chance to discover the source of the scourge that had ravaged the town, so that it could not happen again, anywhere.

In addition to being a man of resolve, M. Delacquis was a man of intense and compassionate sensitivity to the tragedy of the event. The poems and songs that he had written expressed quite eloquently some of these qualities:

> Sadness of a too pure, beautiful morning.
> Sadness still of a sweet summer evening,
> Full of listlessness and murmurs.
> Sadness of being and of having been.
>
> Sadness, light and gray ash
> Which comes down on the ill-understood soul.
> Thou which gives the appearance of death
> To everything that lives, to everything that sleeps.
>
> Sadness, sadness, thou, my friend,
> Sadness of yesterday, sadness of tomorrow,
> My unique treasure, infinite pain.
>
> Be charitable, extend your hand to me.
> With you, my fate will be sweet.
> I want to follow you, anywhere.

But M. Delacquis's own form of sadness did not hinder his resolve. It was he who left his sickbed the moment he could shakily walk, who organized the first meeting of the new association, who brought together the townspeople, the doctors, the authorities of the town, the farmers, the vine tenders, the laborers and their families, to begin the fight for justice and compensation.

Writing to the mayor when he first learned of the interest in forming the association, M. Delacquis said:

> Permit me before anything else to add my congratulations and my thanks to that of the others for the exemplary composure and the total devotion with which you have carried on in the face of recent events.
>
> I join without reservation in your idea to unite in an organization those who in greater or lesser degree have suffered mentally and physically from the acts of negligence of which we have become victims.

Besides the arrests that have already been made, it is essential to continue searching for, and to punish, the perpetrators for whom the lives of men count less than those of cattle and also the public officials whose incompetence and heedlessness are revealed this time as not only ridiculous, but criminal.

It is essential to put an end to an absurd organization [the Union Meunière] which, while it takes the full harvests of grain out of the Midi to supply (so they say) the rest of France, sends to us the scraps of grain from the North and the Center. Is the health of the French there more important than the French here in Gard or in Bouches-du-Rhône?

It is essential that compensation be made for the damages already caused and that we be protected from a recurrence of this event.

No one is able to state positively that recovery will be total. In a few months or a few years organic lesions having their origin in this poisoning can arise and threaten the health, if not the very life, of the victims. With the families who have faced misfortune, I have confidence that you will bring the truth to light in both word and deed.

I put myself at your disposal for any assistance you may demand of me, and which you judge in any way useful.

They met, late in September of 1951, in the upstairs hall of the Café du Luxembourg, on the place de la République, at six in the evening. It was a sad and pathetic group, the halt leading the blind, burning with indignation, steeped in sorrow, crippled by horrifying memories, lost in the confusion about what to do and how to do it. The authorities were there, and Mayor Hebrard accepted the post of honorary president; Dr. Vieu, still drawn and haggard himself, assumed the post of president. Dr. Gabbai was there, barely recovered from his severe setback. Dr. Channac, still far from well, and still bearing the burden of the nights and days without sleep which all the doctors had shared with the victims joined the others.

M. Delacquis, shaky and barely able to stand for more than a few minutes at a time, was elected secretary-general of the association.

Unanimously, the group voted to extend their thanks for the tireless work of the mayor and the doctors who had sacrificed so much for them. They formally expressed equal gratitude to Dr.

Recordier, from Marseilles, and Dr. Giraud and Dr. Latour from Montpellier, as well as the interns from Nîmes, from Avignon, from Montpellier.

Ideas and suggestions were encouraged. M. Delacquis was assigned the job of finding the best possible lawyer in Paris, and M. Moulin, the job of delivering the letter of request personally in Paris. The officers were duly elected, with M. Moulin, the Widow Mison, and the mayor of Carsan all becoming vice presidents. M. Carle, still confined to his bed, was named treasurer. M. le Général de Philip, *conseiller général* of the region, accepted the post of co-honorary president along with Mayor Hebrard. His first act was to suggest that a list be made of the victims of the disaster, especially those who might have need of immediate relief.

There was pathos in the name the victims chose for their organization, as the battle for elusive justice was prepared to launch: *The Association for the Defense of the Victims of the Poisoning by the Bread of Pont-Saint-Esprit* [Gard]. It was an awkward title, but a valid one. They promptly dubbed themselves informally the *Société des Fadas,* the "Society of the not all there"—the one note of humor that came out that evening. There was hope that at least some part of their long days of suffering and lost income would be compensated, and there was action stirring in the wind. A small rubber stamp, the sole asset of the association, was ordered. It required three lines of type face and would be used with firmness and resolve each time M. Delacquis sent forth what was to become a massive and unrelenting flood of letters over the years. It represented the only tangible, material symbol of the group, in the morass of obscurity and mystery that surrounded the case. But to the tired, the drawn, the bent, and the weary it became a blazing escutcheon that would bring them redress from an unthinkable tragedy.

The statutes of the organization were simple; the objectives were to prevent such a disaster from happening again, to determine the responsibility, to see that reparations for damages were justly made, and to provide a reserve pension for those who were thought to be cured, but who might suffer serious relapses. Only those who were medically certified could be admitted, and the annual dues were set at one hundred old francs, or about twenty-five cents. No political or religious discussion would be permitted at any meeting, and anyone who made any fraudulent claims would have his membership immediately terminated. The duration of the association was to be unlimited.

Weak as he was, M. Delacquis lost no time beginning the battle. The burden of the job would fall on his shoulders, and he accepted it without flinching.

The first order of business was to obtain the services of a capable and distinguished lawyer. Mayor Hebrard had already been in touch with a leading attorney in Nîmes, M. Edgar Tailhades, who was both mayor of the city and a senator of the département du Gard. He was willing to collaborate with any Paris expert the association obtained. M. V. de Moro-Giafferri, whose legal activities on behalf of the underdog were known throughout the country, was highly recommended. M. Delacquis, in his first official act as secretary-general of the new organization, wrote him in the name of the president:

> The tragedy of the "bread that kills" has been so thoroughly made known to the public that it is unnecessary for us to recall the manner in which this sad affair has unfolded.
>
> Nearly three hundred sick, five dead, dozens hospitalized in grave condition, many so hopelessly demented that it is not certain whether they will ever regain their reason, families in mourning—such is the balance sheet.
>
> The survivors remain under the menace of a recurrence that might at any time be fatal. We think that your great talents will be of inestimable help to our association. In the name of all the victims we ask you to accept the task of pleading our cause before the court.
>
> Never has the role of an advocate "to defend the widow and the orphan" been so consecrated. We ask that those at fault or the criminals, if there are any, be discovered and punished. We ask that the damages caused by this accident be repaired and that this misery be prevented from happening again in the future, so that others may be spared from suffering as we have suffered and as we are still suffering.
>
> Is there any need to point out that the poisonings have struck, for the most part, the laborers and the small farmers who can least afford it?
>
> Convinced that you will accept the charge that we pray you to accept, we also ask you to be assured of our deepest respect.

As he dictated the letter to Mlle. Wullschleger, she nodded in agreement. She typed the letter carefully, marking well the punctuation and spelling, and carefully pressed the rubber stamp at the top of the sheet of paper when it was finished. No lawyer, she was thinking—however great, however well known in Paris—could fail to respond favorably to such an eloquent appeal. He would carry the hopes of hundreds of people with him as he pleaded at the bar. She personally took the letter to the P.T.T. and posted it in the slot. With the hopes of so many people depending on it, it was worth all her attention.

Meanwhile, there was a great deal of work to do. The names, addresses, ailments, disability, and lost time and wages of all those who sought to join the association had to be registered. Every sickness or disability had to be confirmed as having been actually caused by *le pain maudit* and not by some previous and lingering illness that was unrelated to the current tragedy. It was necessary to register the name of the association officially, to try to obtain funds, and to coordinate medical examinations and medical certifications by the still-exhausted doctors of the village. There were pleas for aid to be made to persons in and outside of Pont-Saint-Esprit, and arrangements for the most needy to try to obtain immediate relief from the proper agencies had to be completed.

M. Delacquis—weak, still trembling from his affliction, with the sight of one eye rapidly deteriorating, and with his voice badly hampered as a result of his suffering—hardly presented an impressive physical appearance. His visage still showed, in spite of its paleness, the lines and well-chiseled planes of a handsome and determined face. From an inner source he summoned the strength to carry out his duties, which were overwhelming enough for a man in the best of physical condition. He conferred at the bedside of M. Carle, who was still unable to walk with any kind of stability, and the two of them agreed to pay out of their own pockets whatever expenses were necessary to launch the attack. Within two days M. Delacquis was able to forward medically certified dossiers to the social security office in Nîmes and to provide General de Philip with a list of those victims whose poverty put them in the status of *premier urgence*.

There was also a necessity to make their cause known to the rest of the country and anywhere else where aid might be forthcoming. M. Delacquis wrote on October 3 to the director of the Reuters news agency:

> I have been informed that one of your journalists visited Pont-Saint-Esprit at the time of the most tragic outbreak of poisonings and offered to aid us in publicizing this unfortunate catastrophe. Since that date, we have formed an association, with the essential objectives of bringing to light the real causes of this mass poisoning and of discovering those responsible, so that the victims who have suffered so much might be indemnified. The families in mourning, the demented still in cells, the sick in danger of a relapse at any time—this is what we are faced with.
>
> Neither the silence that seems to have enveloped the affair nor the inertia of some of the public officials will prevent us from pursuing the objectives that we have undertaken to achieve.
>
> In a few days, our association will be official, and legally recognized.
>
> Our task then will be to aid the press by supplying accurate information, and perhaps to find a means through the press to make a public plea for help. . . .

Although he was a proud man, M. Delacquis knew that in this situation the association would have to beg, and he would not hesitate to do so if it would advance the cause. As he had slowly returned to his senses after the long days and nights of suffering and hallucinations, Mme. Testevin had finally brought him the newspapers he had so persistently demanded. Up until this time, all through his illness, he had had no knowledge of the wide extent of the damage, or of the fact that so many had died or been taken to the psychiatric hospitals.

He had read the papers at a single sitting, shocked and stunned at the succession of events that had been unfolding while he lay in his room. He had read every line, saddened and angered by what had been happening to the villagers, many of whom he knew and loved. Already, it had been growing on him that indemnification was the only form of justice that would count. But he had had no idea of the appalling amount of damage that had been wreaked by the tragedy. His sense of justice, always strong in normal times, was inflamed by the time he had finished reading the papers. The reports instilled in him a quiet and determined form of fury. From it, he gained the strength that now enabled him to summon his energies in the face of his physical weakness.

He was convinced, along with most of the other members of the association, that their case would be infinitely strengthened if a man of de Moro-Giafferri's stature accepted it. He also knew that the famous Paris barrister was in great demand, and that he might not be interested in coming south to the Midi in the face of his heavy work load. What is more, it was necessary to press the civil cases for indemnification with the utmost possible speed. Delays in the acceptance of the case by a lawyer would be added to the endless delays of the court. Meanwhile, people would be facing severe financial problems through their long disabilities and sufferings, both from medical expense and lack of wages. Although M. Tailhades, the Nîmes attorney, had already accepted, would the Paris lawyer be willing to work with him?

It was therefore with the greatest of joy and relief that M. Delacquis opened a letter from M. de Moro-Giafferri that arrived in the first week in October. "I accept willingly with my friend M. Tailhades, the defense of the interests of the victims of Pont-Saint-Esprit, in whose name you have written me. I will put myself immediately in touch with M. Tailhades."

Meanwhile, the most urgent cases could not wait for the ponderous machinery of litigation. The officers of the association jointly appealed to the prefect of Gard to supply immediate emergency aid to over one hundred families who had lost approximately fifty days of work each, a loss that, as ordinary laborers, they could not afford. The officers estimated that a total sum of three million old francs was needed for mere sustenance. This equaled some six thousand dollars, or approximately twenty dollars per victim. The association further warned the prefect that any of those who had been seriously ill could not by any means be considered cured. There were many who wondered why the prefect had not taken any emergency action on his own initiative.

Momentum was gaining, the work toward the objectives proceeding on schedule. In their lack of experience in this kind of process, the victims were unaware of the shoals that lay ahead of them, which would require endless attention to piloting. The first appeared when it was discovered that an association of their classification was not permitted to bring a civil suit before the courts, and that the victims would have to present their cases individually. M. Delacquis quickly dispatched a letter to M. de Moro-Giafferri for advice on this question, and turned his attention to the emergency relief work that General de Philip was conducting through the prefect's office in Nîmes. The progress was both encouraging and discouraging. Social security would cover much of the hospital and medical expenses for those who were eligible, and the majority of the families were. The cases of extreme emergency were allowed three thousand old francs for each family—the sum of six dollars each. The assembly of the *département* of Gard, lacking specific budget and funds to provide more relief, voted to request that the prefect invite all the *communes* of the *département* to solicit funds for the aid of the victims of Pont-Saint-Esprit. The progress was slight and ineffectual, but there was the promise of more assistance if it could be organized and mustered.

The common resolve bound together a widely divergent group of personalities. Their purpose was firm, but they had little else in common but the sorrow and the agony they had been through. Since nothing is more adhesive than a common enemy, their concerted action was without discord at the beginning. But as is true with most groups, minor irritations and abrasions began coming to the forefront soon after the group was organized. One member planned a party at which admission would be charged for the benefit of the victims. Although this was an independent gesture, it fell on the overworked shoulders of M. Delacquis to explain to the other officials, who found this in bad taste, that he had nothing to do with the idea. He reminded them sharply that he had accepted the burdensome job as secretary-general without soliciting it. He was further irritated by the fact that he had heard nothing from M. de Moro-Giafferri since their last request for advice, and M. Delacquis was constantly being pressed by the victims and their families for specific news of the legal progress the association was making. Writing again to the lawyer in Paris, he said:

> Since I have not received any response from my letter of ten days ago, please permit me to point out that we are unable to provide any information to the victims and their families, who question us each day.

> As you can well imagine, they are disturbed by the rumors that are circulating, and they fear that the case is being suppressed; a single word from you, however, will suffice to dissipate all these misunderstandings.
>
> A number of victims have the conviction that, for reasons unknown, the official inquiry is not being conducted in the way that it should. They imagine the worst: the samples of the bread and the flour were confiscated too late, the warehouses and bakeries should have been closed sooner than they were, the official orders to do so were slow in being executed.
>
> You must understand, Sir, our state of mind, and hoping that you will bring us the assistance and the light we need, we pray that you will accept the expression of our respectful sentiments.

While M. Delacquis impatiently awaited a reply, the lawyers for M. Maillet and M. Bruère continued to work for their freedom. Although their first plea had been turned down by the examining magistrate, the second bore fruit. They were released on provisional liberty at the end of October, 1951, after nearly two months in the gloomy prison at Nîmes. In his cell Maillet had cried and suffered atrocious nightmares, in which the people who had died or were rendered insane rose up to speak to him. Timid, frightened, and a pathetic sight in his beret and vest, he left the jail with Bruère. Judge Perrier, now back on the case, was averse to the idea of putting the men on provisional liberty, but the chain of proof and circumstance was thin and tenuous, and a direct link between the disaster at Pont-Saint-Esprit and the actions of the men had not been established. There was only evidence that both of the men had engaged in *fraude alimentaire*. This alone, without being proved that it was connected causally with Pont-Saint-Esprit, took the case out of the hands of Nîmes, and returned it to Vienne, where the men lived and worked.

"We are innocent, that I know for certain," said Bruère to the reporters who greeted them on the steps of the prison. "Nothing is proved against us. We are going to return to Vienne, where we will be judged as the men we are. The one thing I know for sure is that all during the time we have been imprisoned, my bakery has not known any loss of sales whatever. People have signed petitions for us, and have attested to our honor."

Confronted by a reporter with a question about his admitting he had lied to *Commissaire* Sigaud in his questioning, Maillet replied: "That is just not true. They made me say what did not actually happen. I have never made any flour that kills, or that drives people mad!"

At the station they took the train for Bordeaux and Poitiers. Stepping down from their *wagon* they were greeted by their wives and the presidents of both the bakers' and millers' syndicates, and embraced affectionately by both. It was a warm and comforting welcome, but pale beside the scene that greeted them when they arrived in their little village of Saint-Martin-la-Rivière. Nearly two thousand citizens waited for them in the public square, opposite the village church. Here, a huge *feu de joie* fed by bundles of faggots and straw burned brightly with enormous flames. There were tears, there were cries, there was applause.

"In all the villages across the face of France," cried one supporter, "the *boulanger* is the first to rise! Long live Bruère! Long live Maillet!"

In the reflections of the flames, the ancient houses and the faces of the townspeople formed a scene that could have been painted by Bruegel. The street market was there too, along with the curé and the mayor, to greet the newly freed men. To them, the *mise en liberté* of the two men was ample proof of their innocence.

"The accusation of the men for the happenings at Pont-Saint-Esprit is an effrontery," said a friend of the men. "There is perhaps fraud concerning the quality of the flour sent to Gard. But that is another affair."

"There *is* ergot in our region," said the mayor of the town, who was also a seedsman, "but in the course of my career, I have never seen an accident of this sort, even benign, at Saint-Martin-la-Rivière. We have been asked to search for ergot. All the *cultivateurs* have paused in their work, and after several days, one has come to find only a little handful of this parasite. Then why and how, suddenly, is it found in deadly quantity in only a few sacks?"

His was not the only mind on which this question weighed. It weighed on those of the doctors, the *juge d'instruction,* or examining magistrate, the *police judiciaire,* the toxicologists, the doctors, and the layman. It was to become the biggest question of the entire search for reality.

But this and other questions were put aside for the most impressive portion of the welcoming ritual. On the morning of November 6, 1951, the Union Meunière of the *département* of Vienne held a regular meeting in Poitiers, with a special climax planned immediately afterward. At one thirty in the afternoon, the banquet began at the Brasserie de l'Europe. Seated at the table of honor was M. Paul Clement, *président départemental de la Chambre Syndicale de la Meunière,* and he was flanked by M. Maillet and M. Bruère and their wives.

"This poor Maillet," said M. Clement later, "had at last returned to our walls. With my colleagues, we decided to create a thunderous welcoming, a sort of solemn and public rehabilitation. I sent out invitations to authorities and members of the Union Meunière, praying them to give us the honor of their attendance at a banquet given on the return of the Innocents. A grand banquet, no less. The innocence of a man, is that not an occasion for a festival?

"But I had prepared my bombshell, holding back the explosion until the chosen hour. The assemblage arrived at the hotel. A remarkable menu, I should add. We have good palates in our organization. I had previously given my instructions to the waiters: Serve no one until I give the signal!"

M. Clement had instinctive qualities as a showman. As the members filed into the room, seated themselves at the tables, and prepared to eat, he rose and spoke:

"*Messieurs, mesdames,* you do us great honor. Two men who have just come out of prison, who are, in our eyes and yours, innocent, have come here to gain new comfort. Great thanks for that.

"I know, I know that tradition calls for the orations to intervene only at the moment when the champagne sparkles in the goblets. But I have permitted myself to deviate from custom before anything else, to give you this information."

M. Clement paused for effect, and he got it. The audience shifted uneasily in their chairs, vaguely disturbed. M. Clement dramatically looked from face to face, then continued in carefully measured tone.

"Messieurs, the bread that you are about to be served has been made with the flour from Pont-Saint-Esprit. You know—the flour that drives men insane. For my part, I am going to eat all of my share, but you are not obliged to join me. It is then up to your conscience, and I understand it."

He paused again, and after a moment:

"However, I have personally taken all precautions. In a neighboring room, hospital attendants are ready to intervene with strait jackets and stretchers. . . .

"I would like to say to you that the faces of many of our guests seem to have turned a little pale. They are asking themselves if I am joking—or? No, I am not joking, but the hour is not without irony, for I want to make it understood publicly with what extraordinary casualness an innocent man has been thrown in prison."

After a brief comment about justice and the outrages of the magistrate he paused with great solemnity, then said:

"And now—we pass among you at the tables, and eat of the bread made from the flour Maillet supplied to Pont-Saint-Esprit!"

The room was hushed. The *garçons* filed out of the serving pantry with platters of bread. The millers, somewhat shaky and distraught, ate it. And they continued with the rest of the meal, garnished with the full traditions of a French banquet.

When it was over, there were more speeches. M. Pichault, regional president of the Union Meunière, rose and told the gathering what he would have done if he were the police: closed the bakeries earlier, seized the flour, yeast, and salt, searched the premises from top to bottom, nearly all of which the police had done. He continued:

"In spite of all the pressure, the confrontations, the interrogations, our two men, strong in their innocence, refused to acknowledge that they were culpable. During the time, the weeks have been passing, and the toxicologists have scarcely uncovered anything in their research. But it appears more and more improbable that the ergot is at the root of this somber drama.

"In any case, for the eight thousand millers of France, and the fifty thousand *boulangers*, the impossibility of ergot as the cause was clearly untenable from the start, for those who know the commercial milling process."

He wound up his discourse by addressing the *juge d'instruction* of Nîmes, in absentia, directly:

"You are taking a false road, the millers and bakers of Vienne assure you."

There were other talks, mainly from Union Meunière officials or the bakers' associations of the locality. Some said they welcomed the enlightenment of the public about their functions. Nearly all of them said they were convinced the flour from Vienne was not responsible for the tragedy, but they did not articulate just how they were able to know this. Nor did they make any references to the flurry of sicknesses at Connaux and Saint-Génies-de-Comolas prior to the Pont-Saint-Esprit outbreaks.

After the talks were finished, the dishes cleared, the *café filtre* served, the cognac sipped, Maillet rose shyly to thank the gathering, in his name and Bruère's:

"Thank you all in this dolorous situation, for ourselves and our families. Your group has brought us precious moral aid."

The press, hungry for new developments in the situation, gave the event voluminous coverage. One journal sharply rapped the knuckles of the organization sponsoring the banquet by saying: "In spite of the festivities, it is important to remember that the charge of distributing flour unfit for consumption still remains. . . ."

Another journal of the Midi wrote:

> If the millers and bakers of Vienne feel sure that Maillet and Bruère have been wrongly imprisoned, they are free to welcome them warmly. They must not forget, however, that as a result of this affair, there are the dead, the seriously ill, and the afflicted families, who command a measure of decency.

But the gentle and soft-spoken M. Delacquis, along with the members of the association of the victims of *le pain maudit*, read the accounts of the feast, the toasts, the testimonials, and the celebration with utter awe and incredulity. Joining them with the same reaction were Judge Perrier and Commissioner Sigaud.

It did not take long for any of them to go into action.

ELEVEN

M. Delacquis acted first. Trembling as much now from anger as from sickness, he dictated in his weak and hoarse voice a stinging letter to M. Clement, who had opened the festivities with the startling news that the guests were being served bread made from the flour that had been used in Pont-Saint-Esprit.

> The newspapers have brought us the echo of the celebrations and rejoicing that the millers, the bakers, and the farmers of Saint-Martin-la-Rivière believed useful to organize as a welcome for their "martyrs," Messieurs Maillet and Bruère. We would have believed it to be a journalist's joke, if the same newspapers had not confirmed the facts the next day.
>
> We think that the producers of rye who carried to the baker the sweepings of their grain and took the good flour in exchange have some reason to thank their compatriots for not having eaten their own flour. But we also think that their gratitude could manifest itself with less fanfare and without insults to the victims of Pont-Saint-Esprit.
>
> The affair that has amused you so much and that has caused the spiritual director of the mills of Villards to say, "The crazier you are, the more you laugh," has actually caused some rather deplora-

ble consequences: five dead and two hundred so badly stricken that their health is seriously damaged and they can find no repose and no happiness. These are, in our opinion, realities that command a little decency, if not respect.

Perhaps our judgment appears false to you and will give you more reason to believe in our insanity and in our laughter. However, if you wish to see some of the objects of your amusement, why not come here yourself? To provoke among your compatriots the most wholesome hilarity there are in the hospital at Nîmes two mothers, one with five children and the other with two, who are behind bars and tied down to their beds for most of the time. They do not recognize either their children or their husbands and laugh nearly all the time, without cease.

In the name of the members of our association, I hope you will convey our thanks to all those among you who were so kind as to think of us and to speak of us with such emotion. We regret only that we are not rich enough to go to you and express our gratitude in person and have you witness our condition.

We would be very much obliged if you would read our letter to your adherents and to the generous population of Saint-Martin-la-Rivière, and we would be fools of joy if you would give it to the publisher of your newspaper in Vienne.

Counting, in spite of all, on your spirit of equity, we pray you to accept, Monsieur, our distinguished sentiments.

Judge Perrier reacted differently, but just as sharply.

If M. Clement *had* furnished the flour for the bread eaten at the banquet from the stock of flour used for the bread causing the tragedy at Pont-Saint-Esprit, where did he get it? All the flour in the region from that time period had been seized and was either under official seal or in the laboratories.

In a grim official communiqué to the chief of the Seventeenth Brigade of the *police judiciaire* M. Perrier asked that M. Clement be questioned on whether he had obtained such flour, and if so, from where and on what date. The judge also wanted to know who had taken it, who had transported it, and who had made the bread.

At his interrogation by the police, M. Clement was considerably less voluble than at the banquet. He admitted that he had organized the banquet for the two men upon their release from prison, and that they had nothing to do with it. He admitted that he had said that the bread was made of flour Maillet had furnished Pont-Saint-Esprit, and that it would be passed to the tables. But he claimed that he said this only because someone at the gathering had suggested this to him during the course of the earlier meeting of the Union Meunière, and that it was just a comment arising from a private conversation. He could not recall who it was that suggested it. Actually, the bread was supplied and served by the restaurant, and he had no idea whatever from where it came. The manager of the restaurant, in turn, admitted that the bread was that of his regular supplier in the area, and that M. Clement's statements were the result of "pure fantasy."

Fantasy or not, the episode in the Brasserie de l'Europe did nothing to endear the Union Meunière to the victims. It did, however, serve to change the mood of the association from that of sorrow to that of anger—blazing anger. The preoccupation with sickness and death shifted to the search for the truth, the source, the cause, in spite of the fact that dozens remained seriously ill and several remained in or were returned to the psychiatric cells of the hospital. It became a passion with M. Delacquis, never a patient man, who smarted under what he felt was gross injustice. The delays, the slowness of the inquiry, the failure to see any direct action from his own attorneys, were frustrating and agonizing. The pressure from the members of the association for action was constant, and combined with the seeming lack of action on the part of the officials, M. Delacquis found himself in a vise whose pressure increased with his own swollen anger. "No response has been received from two letters to M. de Moro-Giafferri," he wrote to the lawyer in Nîmes, "and we are faced with the impossibility of satisfying the numerous demands for information that are made by the stricken." He went on to say that the association had not even been officially registered, although nearly three weeks had passed.

There were some bright shafts of hope. The Municipal Council of Alès, a town whose history went back to the Phocaeans and whose streets and *allées* had been struck with a series of massive plagues in the 1840's, until Pasteur made his pioneering discoveries there, voted to send the association at Pont-Saint-Esprit fifty thousand old francs as an expression of sympathy. And although this sum amounted to only one hundred dollars, it bolstered the spirits of the villagers and gave them faith that others were sympathetic to their plight. It did nothing, however, to soothe M. Delacquis's inquietude about the silence that had descended upon the case. A month had gone by after his second letter to the Paris lawyer, and he wrote again: "We do not understand why our progress seems to be at a dead standstill after three months. The victims urgently need both material help and a knowledge of the truth. We are persuaded that you understand the state of our minds, and that you will intervene quickly on our behalf."

But the formation of the association seemed to add another dimension to a case in which everyone concerned was continuing to fight against elusive phantoms. Nothing could be pinned down. The ghost was everywhere—and nowhere. The police probed and seemed to be reaching a conclusive assembly of evidence, only to see it dissolve in front of their eyes. The doctors fought against symptoms that responded to nothing. The victims struck out with hope and energy, only to find that they seemed to be shadow boxing. The toxicologists found ergot in some cases, but in extremely small quantities. They encountered mysterious and unidentified alkaloids with it, but nowhere, even when the ergot was present, did there seem to be enough quantity to cause the lethal, massive concentrations that could flatten hundreds of people.

The most sober and most intelligent of the investigators agreed that the affair was something no one wanted to happen, that it was accidental, and that no criminal action was involved. Maillet and Bruère certainly had no intention or thought of creating such a tragedy, even if they had engaged in some improper practices. M. Briand would not want to ruin his business, his reputation, and his standing in the community. The Union Meunière, in spite of its indifference and even callous disregard in compensating the victims, would have no desire to expose itself to litigation which was bound to ensue. Even the most insane criminal would be totally unlikely to find a poison that could elude modern medicine, and which would be administered so clumsily and haphazardly. It was a drama without a villain, except for the phantom that continued to hover over the village on the Rhône—an unknown, unrecognizable, and unidentified phantom which was impervious to the slings and arrows of the outraged victims, the test tubes of the laboratories, the syringes of the doctors, the handcuffs of the police, the briefs of the lawyers, and the strait jackets of the orderlies.

Impatience was another villain, too. It infected the police, the victims, and the laboratories, and although it was understandable and perhaps inevitable in the conditions that existed, it measurably hindered the progress of the case, frayed nerves, and served no one. The impatience of M. Delacquis was sincere and was a result of righteous indignation, but it was sometimes misplaced. He failed to follow proper channels at times, drawing anger and irritation from some officials who were trying to help. He was rebuked by the *conseiller général* and the mayor for it because they themselves were impatient, but they knew that the machinery moved more slowly than desired. They also knew that practically nothing could be done about it.

M. Delacquis's impatience about the slowness of the registration of the association was mollified when the prefect of Gard himself, who is equivalent to the governor of a state, received a delegation of members of the association and revealed to them that he himself had thought of the idea of an association being formed. The meeting did much to dissipate the feeling among the victims that the state was covering up and smothering the case.

But the slowness on the part of the lawyers to advise the association on what steps to take still continued to rankle, as well as the lack of any specific material succor for the stricken.

M. Tailhades, responding to one of M. Delacquis's letters of inquiry about all this, wrote on December 11 to say that he understood the concern expressed, but that the process would necessarily be slow. "I saw M. de Moro-Giafferri on my last visit to Paris," the Nîmes lawyer wrote, "and he was astonished that he had not replied to your letters." M. Delacquis noted with some irony that this seemed odd to him, that a man should be astonished by his own lack of reply to routine correspondence. But he was pleased that at least the two men had met and seemed to be planning some action, vague as it was. All through October and November he had received a constant stream of the sick and their families in his office at the Coopérative des Céréales, and all during those weeks he was wearied by trying to explain to them the reasons for the delay, of which he was not sure himself. As his strength returned with infinite slowness, the vision in his left eye was rapidly deteriorating, the result of cardiovascular ravages of the plague, which had created severe damage to the retinal artery. The prognosis was not good, and it weighed constantly on his mind. It did not, however, diminish his resolve. It did, in fact, spur him on to more action.

There were endless details to assess, assemble, and appraise. There was the request by Mme. Briand to join the association, when it was becoming apparent that the association would be forced, technically at least, to bring the suits for civil damages against M. Briand himself. He in turn would have to seek redress from the Union Meunière, as suppliers and distributors of the flour.

There was the expediting of the emergency aid promised by the prefecture, which was not only infinitely small, but would require a month's delay before the payments would be made. A delay of a month in the sending of the funds "for the relief of the poor people who suffer still from the effects of the poisoning" was unthinkable, M. Delacquis wrote, adding: "It seems to us that in this occurrence, a little humanity ought to have precedence over *les chinoiseries bureaucratiques*. We count absolutely on your spirit of understanding for the necessity of providing the funds before the end of the week. In case of a contrary response, we will address ourselves to those whose voice will be susceptible of being better heard than ours."

M. Delacquis, in spite of his attempts to keep his anger down, found that the constant stream of irritations caused him to flare up at the least provocation. Each night when he returned to La Villette he would see the drawn and pinched features of M. Testevin's once-handsome face, the limping shakiness of Mme. Dezeuzes, the exhaustion of Mme. Testevin—and Emile.

Emile had just returned from the hospital. He was almost a twisted skeleton. His frame was bent and his features contorted. He needed constant care. Of all those at La Villette, he had suffered the most. Yet his spirit was buoyant and resilient. He refused to admit that he could not regain his strength, and he followed the routine prescribed by Dr. Gabbai relentlessly. Looking at Emile through his reduced and hampered vision, M. Delacquis's resolve was nourished and made stronger each day. And it was further buttressed by a letter received from Mme. Félix

Mison, widow of the first person to have died. In February, 1952, she wrote M. Delacquis:

"Not being able to continue to live alone in the farm of my husband Félix, it has been necessary for me to leave Carsan and to live with friends here at Istres, in the Bouches-du-Rhône. I would be very grateful if you would let me know if you have been supplied with all the necessary medical information to establish the proper dossier for the association. . . ."

Mme. Mison's letter would go unanswered by M. Delacquis personally. For the strain, the effort, the pressures of the work for both the association and the cooperative were too much for him, and he fell into a serious relapse which sent him reeling back to his bed at La Villette.

So intensely was the focus of the village centered on the unraveling of the mystery of the plague, that two tragic events passed by without broad notice throughout France. Mme. Carle, the mother of M. Carle, died, with her death hastened by the poisoning, and M. Guigou the *pensionnaire* of the Hôtel Redortier, who had ironically brought his own bread to the table there, also became a fatal victim. The toll had now mounted to seven deaths, but the laboratories seemed no nearer a definitive appraisal of the cause than they were in the beginning.

The doctors, under the guidance of Professor Giraud and Professor Latour of Montpellier, had joined together to assemble a massive report for the French academy of medicine on the subject, and were working on it independently of both the police and the toxicologists. There did not seem to be any overt conflict between the two teams of professional men, but there did seem to be obscure smolderings to indicate there was some under the surface. It was rumored about the village that the doctors were not pleased with the way the laboratory analysis was going, that many of the medical men felt that an undefined *raison d'état* was at work to slow down the investigation, a covering up for somebody, an intervention somewhere by *des hommes politiques* which was blocking the work at the laboratories.

If there were such manipulations going on, there was certainly no evidence that the police were not prosecuting the case fully. The dossiers were growing fatter daily, the detectives taking infinite pains to track down every possible clue.

Judge Perrier, smarting under the criticism in the press about the apparent slowness of the over-all investigation prepared a *commission rogatoire* for *le capitaine de gendarmerie* at Uzès to investigate this possibility fully.

"Certain journals," he wrote to the captain, "have recently published some articles relative to the poisonings of Pont-St.-Esprit, saying that the *gendarmerie* possesses some information which would name those responsible for the tragedy, and accusing the *police judiciaire* of having oriented the research in the wrong direction.

"Without adding fuel to this twaddle, I would like you to inform me if the *gendarmerie* is in possession of any information that could not be verified and exploited by the *police judiciaire*. If the answer is affirmative, I would appreciate your giving me the details, and I would like to hear any useful witnesses.

"There is even a rumor that there is another death. If this is correct, invite the parents to produce a certificate of death and a medical certificate attesting that the death is caused by a poisoning."

Another rumor circulating at high velocity was that the Union Meunière, faced with the possibility of overwhelming and shattering civil damages, was doing everything in its power to shift the responsibility to the baker, the transport system, or any other possible place. The statements and attitude of the Union Meunière officials at the banquet for Maillet and Bruère did nothing to enhance its reputation in the eyes of anyone concerned. If anything, the result was to intensify the efforts of Judge Perrier and Commissioner Sigaud to press the inquiry further into the flour milled by Maillet.

Nearly all of Maillet's supply of flour made during the period under observation had been shipped out of Vienne to the Pont-Saint-Esprit area. All of this was being subjected to the toxicological tests at Marseille. One shipment of Maillet to a baker in his own region went to M. Payrault in the village of Tercé, in Vienne. The tests on this and on the other samples taken from the Pont-Saint-Esprit area were not encouraging from Maillet's point of view. Of 113 samples 99 were declared unfit for consumption. Specifically, samples #266 and #415, from the shop of M. Payrault in Tercé, were found to be lethal in tests on sixty white mice over a period of several months. In addition, the tests showed that

5 percent of the flour was made from rye and that ergot was present at the rate of one unit per thousand. But here was the exasperating problem again: This amount of ergot was assumed to be negligible from the toxicological point of view. Whether this concentration had been stronger at an earlier date and had chemically deteriorated since then was impossible to tell. Yet even with this minimum concentration, the mice had died. This paradox was only increased when Maillet, after he was confronted by Commissioner Sigaud with the results of the tests, demanded that other experts confirm the results. Maillet named the director of the laboratories of the millers' school of France, and the court named the head of the laboratory for the investigation of frauds at Paris. The results later turned out to be inconclusive and contradictory and did nothing to either advance or injure Maillet's case. In the eyes of the Nîmes officials Maillet remained guilty of *fraude alimentaire,* but no causal chain could be established with the Pont-Saint-Esprit tragedy, and the case was no longer within the jurisdiction of the département du Gard.

Meanwhile, M. Delacquis had recovered from his relapse and was still trying to obtain some kind of word from M. de Moro-Giafferri, the association's own attorney. To the distraught secretary-general of the organization, it was incredible that a lawyer who had agreed to take on a case would not write him and advise him of any developments and instruct him what to do. The Paris lawyer had confirmed his acceptance of the case the first week in October of 1951. By the middle of March, 1952, some six months later, M. Delacquis had had no direct word. He was embarrassed by the constant inquiries of the victims who asked him what was being done to help their serious financial and medical stress. Grasping at straws, M. Delacquis learned that a lawyer in Valence whom he knew slightly would see Moro-Giafferri in that city, and he wrote a note on March 18 asking him to pass along an urgent request for some kind of action. M. Delacquis desperately hoped that the letter to Moro-Giafferri would be personally handed to him:

> Slowly but surely, an enormous silence settles around our affair. The laboratories are strangely silent, the police investigation seems to suffer from foot-rot, and the unfortunate victims of Pont-Saint-

Esprit, who continue to bear their sufferings from the poisoning of August, 1951, along with the families in mourning, who cannot forget their dead, are more and more under the anguished impression that the men charged with bringing light to the affair are, quite frankly, obeying orders to stifle the inquiry.

We are, however, among those who still believe in the justice of man, and we hope for the day when those responsible will be known and the damages caused will be repaired.

I reiterate to you, Maître, that we have placed our confidence and our hope in you, and that we will be heartbroken if you must, for motives that we know not, also observe the law of silence.

We think that it would be possible to rouse and stir the toxicologists assigned by the examining magistrate, who have been dawdling before us for seven months. These delays are inadmissible. It is not a question of some mere financial scandal, but of an affair that has resulted in seven deaths, sick who are incapable of resuming their work, and whose families are plunged into misery, and human beings by the dozens who no longer have faith in anything, and who are near revolt.

That is why I am permitting myself to approach you on the occasion of your visit to Valence and to address this letter to you through a friend, who has kindly agreed to give this letter to you. I hope that within the next day we may have the truth.

It was a desperate letter, and M. Delacquis knew it. But he had almost reached the end of his patience, and his own illness, accompanied by the fading vision in his eye, drove him to extraordinary despair.

Within two days he received a letter from his friend, with the dismal news that Moro-Giafferri's case in Valence had been postponed for at least two months and asking if M. Delacquis wanted the letter forwarded to Paris or held until that time. Glumly recognizing the lack of response his letters to Paris had received, M. Delacquis suggested that his friend hold the letter until May 6, the new date of Moro-Giafferri's arrival.

Meanwhile, he turned his attention to the emergency aid from the *département*. A total of seven hundred dollars had been voted by the municipalities of Gard as aid to the victims. The *département* itself had further allocated an average payment of about thirty-five dollars per victim as a stopgap measure. Only about ten dollars of this amount had been actually paid to each victim, and none of the voluntary contributions had been received at all. In a statement prepared at a meeting at the Café du Luxembourg on April 26, 1952, the association expressed its feelings:

> The poisoned victims of Pont-Saint-Esprit, after holding a general meeting on April 26, 1952, at which they were informed of the progress of their case as regards both the investigation and the distribution of aid, confirm the following statements:
>
> 1. After seven months the laboratories have not yet given their opinion on the cause of the poisonings.
> 2. The humanitarian gestures previously made by the state, the *département*, and the municipalities have not been tangibly followed up by the distribution of the money that has been offered and allocated.
>
> They ask that the deputies of the National Assembly
>
> —Intervene with great energy in the Assembly to demand that the laboratories immediately give their official opinion.
> —Direct a serious inquiry entirely free of all political considerations to seek out those who are responsible, and to determine the responsibility of each.
> —Direct that all allocated funds be immediately distributed to the victims.

By the end of April this statement went out in the form of a letter to all members of the National Assembly from the *département* of Gard, signed by Dr. Vieu, president of the association.

The deputies replied promptly and sympathetically. They agreed, almost unanimously that the funds should be distributed. The results of their response would not be known for some time, but at least one concrete development happened. An anonymous donor from the town of Alès sent over fifty cents in stamps as a contribution.

Monsieur le Général de Philip pleaded eloquently in the meetings of the General Council of Gard.

But astonishingly little happened to clarify the thick cloud of obscurity that surrounded the case.

The doctors who had worked at the bedsides of the *malades*

were by now convinced, however, that the symptoms they had encountered, analyzed, tabulated, and appraised could only be attributed to one thing: Ergotism. The report to the French Academy of Medicine was now almost complete, the combined efforts of the doctors Giraud and Latour of Montpellier, along with their interns, Lisbonne and Pourquier; Channac, Gabbai, and Vieu of Pont-Saint-Esprit; Pitot and Meissonnier, of the hospital at Nîmes; Martin, Amphoux, and Vincent of l'Hôpital Psychiatrique de Font-d'Aurelle in Montpellier; Sarran, of *des hôpitaux* d'Avignon; Suttel, and Dussot, of the Hôpital Psychiatrique de Montdevergues, and their interns, Maubert, Dumas, and Ratehdra.

They formed a firm and combined front with the theory that ergot was at the base of the poisonings, in spite of the protestations that the concentrations of ergot already found in the samples and viscera did not show evidence that there was enough concentration and quantity of the poison to do the massive damage that had followed in the wake of the "accursed bread." They also stood firm against the protests of the Union Meunière that the bread would have been uneatable and black if ergot had been the cause.

One outspoken doctor wrote to Judge Perrier on April 29, 1952:

> I have read during the past few days the communication that Professor Giraud of Montpellier has prepared for the National Academy of Medicine on the poisonings of Pont-Saint-Esprit. As to the nature of the poison, I am only able to go along with Professor Giraud; The clinical symptoms confirmed at the bedsides of the patients are those of *ergot de seigle*. . . .
>
> My impression on the slowness and silence of the laboratories is that they *desire* this, and that the silence is *imposed* by political forces.
>
> Actually, no one is able to affirm if there is any *malade* who is completely cured. I am constantly assisting the sick at frequent, insidious crises that reappear periodically. . . .
>
> P.S. My dear Perrier, I know that you would like this whole mystery clarified, but after seven months I remain skeptical that any discovery will be made of those who are culpable—whether it is the Union Meunière or an individual who committed homicide through carelessness.

The report by the practicing physicians to the French Academy totaled twenty-five thousand words. It examined every facet of their experience with the tragedy. It pointed out that there was no direct correlation between the amount of the bread eaten and the effects, because generally no more than five hundred grams was consumed. It reviewed the symptoms and the stages in which the symptoms developed, and it included a day-by-day breakdown of the progress of the plague as it built to *l'éclosion brutale* on the eighth day. It traced the new symptoms which developed after the twentieth day: the hemorrhages, the gangrene, and the skin eruptions. It detailed the precise physiological symptoms which were correlated with the psychological outbreaks. It charted the results of the electroencephalograph examinations, the cardiograph recordings, the pulse rates, the optical examinations, the blood pressure readings. It noted that no definitive word had been received from the laboratories, although the presence of ergot of cereals was definitely found, as well as several other elusive alkaloids which had not been identified, a common finding where ergot alkaloids were concerned. It emphasized that the doctors were forced to remain in the role of clinicians, analyzing the scene from the point of view of what they had observed in their clinical confrontations, and that whatever origin of the poison was discovered, there should be a correlation between that and the clinical symptoms. It summarized the results to date from the laboratories, which included: (1) That many samples of the bread and flour seized and tested had shown in laboratory tests to be highly toxic to animals, (2) that no mineral poison had been detected, (3) that ergot and unknown alkaloids had been discovered and clearly noted.

The question of how it was possible for ergot in such minimal quantities to create the damage was the main stumbling block of the report, because it was agreed that ergot, per se, could not be so devastating, and that it was used medically, without harm, in doses equal to what must have been absorbed by the victims who had eaten the bread.

Before the full report was completed, there were suspicions growing among the doctors that might be able to explain this anomaly. It had been established that the taste of the bread was good, that there were no real complaints about this from those who had eaten it. The dough, also, had risen normally, cooked well, and except for the slight grayish color to the paste, there had been nothing to indicate that it was suffused with ergot in any great quantity.

In the summer of 1951 there had been many experiments, in process over several previous years, on the properties of ergot, in the hope of finding more useful thereapeutic values to extend its already known value in cases of high blood pressure, migraine headache, birth inducement, and other disorders.

The poison of *le pain maudit* would have to have been practically colorless, tasteless, and incredibly powerful. It would have to have been so concentrated that even a single mouthful of bread containing the tasteless poison would be capable of creating violent illness, and in some cases, death. Even arsenic, the classic poison of history, could not have accomplished this, except over a long period of time. It would also be immediately detectable in any quantity. Insecticides and fungicides were always involved in the growing and protection of foods of every kind, including grain, and there was often the presence of these to a degree in many kinds of foods. But, except under long periods of consumption, these, also, could not logically have created the violent, traumatic psychic outbreak that characterized the "accursed bread." Further, the symptoms would have been different from those revealed by the citizens of Grand Rue and environs. Beyond that, historic ergotism had in the past produced identical symptoms at a time when pesticides were unknown. And although the presence of fungicides and insecticides had not been obvious in the classic toxilogical methods used at the beginning of the laboratory tests, the doctors felt that even if later specific tests revealed the presence of them, this possible cause could be discounted. It would be necessary, for instance, for a person to absorb clearly detectable amounts of an organo-mercurial fungicide to cause the death of a human being, and the flour and bread would be saturated with the coloring agent of the fungicide. Further, the symptoms already considered by the doctors would be measurably different, with disorder, permanent damage, and destruction of the kidney being the classic and key symptom. In the victims of Pont-Saint-Esprit, there was practically no sign of this, nor of the ashen gray color of the mouth. No mercury, further, was discovered in the urine of the *malades*, almost a certainty if even a mildly toxic dose had been absorbed. The other symptoms possible from the ingestion of mercury alkyls sometimes included insomnia and hallucinations, but only from chronic poisoning by small exposures over a long period of years. The ingestion in a single dose did not bring hallucinations, insomnia, or mental trouble. The night of *l'éclosion brutale* in Pont-Saint-Esprit established clearly that the poison of *le pain maudit* was launched in a single, massive dosage in the bread. Further, gangrene was not a symptom of mercury poisoning, even in massive doses. The entire pathological image of the plague simply did not match this possibility. There was no question that the over-all picture matched the sporadic epidemics of the Middle Ages, caused by rye and wheat rot, which in turn caused the growth of the elusive and mystical ergot. But no one had yet, in the course of history, determined just how the ergot was able to do its sweeping damage without being detected by taste and odor at the moment when the victim ate the bread. Ordinary ergot would most certainly cause the consumer to be revolted by it, to spit it out, and to take the bread back to the baker for a new loaf. Even harmless mold on bread causes it to be rejected. Was there something else lurking, something hidden in the mysterious ergot alkaloids, arising spontaneously out of nature, which still resisted identification in the year of 1951? It was known, for instance, that ergot in the natural state was far more powerful and unpredictable than in synthetic form. But from the evidence at hand, both clinically and toxicologically, there was no *widely known and clearly established* poison that could have the characteristic of being tasteless and colorless, powerful enough to ravage nearly three hundred people, concentrated enough to make even small mouthfuls toxic and lethal, and still leave so little toxicological evidence in the bread samples and viscera. Further, the massive and giant hallucinations, breaking out in concert, preceded by the strange state of euphoria, were totally unique in modern toxicology, and could be matched only in the medical histories of the Middle Ages and sporadically in other epochs, when primitive scientists could not analyze or determine what the chemical composition of the poison might be. Further, these historic ravages could not possibly be caused by pesticides or fungicides, since they had not yet been discovered. Neither conventional ergot nor gargantuan doses of insecticides could accomplish these tragic results, even with long-term absorption. With such an unknown poison, Maillet, Bruère, Briand, the Union Meunière, or anyone else who had anything to do with the grain, flour, or bread would be innocent victims of the tragedy, as well as the others. It would be, in effect, a spontaneous and rare act of nature that no one could foretell or foreshadow. There would remain only the technical, legal, and civil responsibility of protecting the consumer from hidden defects, a responsibility remaining with supplier and vendor regardless of the mystery of the source.

When M. Delacquis had bicycled up the hill to La Villette on the tragic day when the sickness struck him, he had reeled dizzily in a world which suddenly had turned into a place where time and dimension contracted and expanded, where colors had taken on an entirely new aura, where his concept of himself and the universe exploded into an inexplicable realm. M. Testevin encountered almost the same phenomenon. When he mounted his bicycle, it spun out from under him as he attempted to keep his balance in a world that seemed to be undergoing a silent earthquake.

Only a few years before the malady struck Pont-Saint-Esprit, a Swiss chemist by the name of Hofmann rode a bicycle home from his work in the laboratoire de Rothlin and had experienced almost the identical reaction. His bicycle twisted and wobbled on the road, and the conventional world went haywire. Along with his colleague, Dr. Stoll, he was working on many experimental studies involving the chemical derivatives of ergot. On this particular day he was working in the obscure netherland of ergot alkaloids, on the track of other useful pharmaceutical applications for the Sandoz Company, one of the leading pharmaceutical companies in the world, based in Switzerland. Arriving at his home, Hofmann not only underwent a strange and utterly fantastic metamorphosis, but he hallucinated and viewed the strangest of sights and the most rare and exotic colors he had ever seen. His horizons contracted and expanded, and he seemed to grow inside himself, later viewed himself from the outside looking in. What was most puzzling was that only a tiny, infinitesimal amount of the alkaloid had touched his lips accidently, a dosage which in terms of ordinary ergot would have been completely unnoticed.

So utterly strange was his experience that, when he recovered, he immediately determined to track down and identify the source of his experience, an experience so shattering he could not describe it in words.

The questions he had were many. How could such a miniscule dosage produce such gargantuan effects? How could it be trapped and separated from the other ergot alkaloids? How could a parasitic fungus that grows on the tips of rye or wheat bring about such a profound change of personality that he was still, several days later, shattered by the experience? What would be the social effects of such a drug? Were there any therapeutic values?

Along with Dr. Stoll, he began his researches, the result of his auto-observation of the effect the drug had on him, personally.

It was not long before the facts began to emerge. From the ergot came lysergic acid. From lysergic acid came the specific form that the source of his poisoning assumed. It was colorless and tasteless. It was among the most powerfully concentrated poisons yet encountered. One *one-hundred-thousandth* of an ounce could cause unbelievable and unpredictable reactions. An eyedropper could contain enough for five thousand doses. A single, effective dose of 250 micrograms would fail to cover the head of a pin. Later, an experimental dose was to kill an elephant. Its lethal power as far as white mice were concerned would turn out to be double that of its parent alkaloid, ergobasine. Its cousins were ergotoxine and ergotamine, whose pronounced effects on the cardiovascular and digestive system were well known and identified. But the new drug's reactions clearly separated it from its relatives. Ergotamine was one of the active principles of ergot, and the new drug was very easily derived from it. The first animal experiments created nervous agitation, extreme salivation, and catatonic rigidity, in addition to death. Pigeons and salamanders struck statue-like poses—or "strutted like penguins." One drop of the drug in a million drops of water set carp into a tailspin. The fur of cats stood on end, and the drug left them with total insomnia. The first experimental oral doses on human beings, including Hofmann himself, confirmed that only an infinitely small amount was necessary to create deep psychic disturbances and hallucinatory delirium, in addition to complete mental confusion. Later, one key reaction was to be observed: The desire to jump from any windowsill that could be found.

These reactions were the result of approximately one two-millionth of a pound of the drug, about equivalent to stirring a single rain drop into a swimming pool. It was to turn out to be so powerful that an effective dose could be painted on a postage stamp or a fingernail.

The physiological effects of large doses on human beings were to remain largely unknown because no chemist would attempt to impose an experiment of this size, with the results almost sure to be disastrous on the basis of animal tests. Of all the derivatives of the ergot alkaloids, the strange new drug brought the most intense reaction, especially in its unique psychic effects, including the vivid visual hallucinations, the brilliant colors, and the general state of euphoria. The luminosity of the colors was perhaps the most pronounced of the early symptoms discovered; then the expansion and contraction of the surroundings, the lack of orientation in time and space. Alternating with euphoria was depression—deep and unrelenting on occasion, with terrifying, maniacal agitation and disorder, incessant talking, long-continued bursts of insane laughter. The experimental subjects, in their stages of *euphorie béate* felt supremely powerful, but were unable to walk or stand correctly, and according to their preexisting tendencies, were at times motivated toward suicide. But the consciousness was retained. The subjects knew they were hallucinating, retaining a large measure of judgment and memory. Often, after taking the new drug, the subject seemed to be looking down and observing himself from the outside. Obsessions, compulsions, and *les idées fixes* often arose. One of the early volunteers tried to jump out of the window to end his compulsion. There was considerable evidence that the subjects showed a total disgust for tobacco. Also revealed was the fact that the experimenters at times encountered an impression that their arms or legs sunk into the body, their heads doing the same, or all members separating from the body. Sexuality played no specific part in the symptoms revealed. Although the drug then in the process of discovery created reactions similar to mescaline, its power in subcutaneous injection was two thousand times as strong. But it differed from mescaline in that it produced no liver damage. In the over-all appraisal it produced above all the extraordinarily rich elementary visual illusions and hallucinations, a rare state of euphoric exaltation, and often horrifying depression.

As a drug, the new and unexpected ergot alkaloid revealed

another quality: It was extremely volatile, soluble in water, and unstable, as were the rest of its ergot family, and would deteriorate chemically so fast that it was often lost from view before some experiments could be completed.

The first studies confirmed that this amazing collection of symptoms following the use of the drug came from the infinitely small dosages. Nobody knew, or wanted to know, what might happen if massive overdoses of the tasteless and odorless drug were absorbed by a broad spectrum of people.

The drug, of course, was lysergic acid diethylamide, or LSD-25.

TWELVE

In August of 1951, when M. Briand mixed his batter, and when M. Delacquis and all the others sat down to eat the bread coming from it, LSD-25 was practically unknown as a hallucinogenic drug. As Hofmann continued working with Stoll, it is reported that both were alarmed and wary of the monster they had accidentally created. When Hofmann and Stoll heard of the poisonings in Pont-Saint-Esprit, they were further alarmed because the psychogenic symptoms were identical to those of LSD-25, and the two of them were sitting on top of the knowledge that the possible explanation for *ergotisme historique* might lie partially in the discovery of the new drug. Could ergot—on rare historic occasions—spontaneously and accidentally form into a particularly potent form of *natural* LSD, thus creating an accidental overdose, which in turn could cause St. Anthony's Fire?

The two men lost no time getting in touch with Professor Giraud at the University of Montpellier, and within days a meeting was held with many of the doctors involved in the Pont-Saint-Esprit case. Hofmann and Stoll revealed their new studies to them, and compared the results to those of *le pain maudit*. They reviewed all the facts together: how ergot forms on rye grain, then ferments under certain conditions of humidity, liberating several alkaloids of ergot. LSD-25, it was noted, was one of the alkaloids produced by the fermentation of ergot. But this spontaneous condition was extremely rare, as the sporadic history of ergotism—St. Anthony's Fire—had shown over the centuries.

Hofmann pulled no punches when he talked to the doctors gathered at Montpellier. He described the discovery of the new drug as "appalling, frightful, and shocking." He told them that, regrettably, if it were improperly used and distributed, it might bring more destruction than the atomic bomb. Highlighting the psychogenic effects of LSD-25 and historical ergotism, which were strikingly similar, he condensed them into two main categories: (1) Magical and enchanting hallucinations of colors, in the nature of an Ali Baba's cave; (2) Atrocious hallucinations, including changes in distances, or with the ceiling descending and the walls closing in on the victim. The new discovery did not produce direct erotic symptoms, as hashish and other drugs often did.

He noted that the alkaloids released by the fermentation of ergot deteriorate chemically in very short order, that the examinations made and being made in the police laboratories would detect few, if any, of the ergot alkaloids, even if they had been present at the beginning.

The doctors at the meeting agreed that mercury poisoning was not evident in any manner, especially because of the persistent lack of kidney or liver damage.

The doctors sensed that, aside from the mystery of the Pont-Saint-Esprit tragedy, they were sitting on the threshold of a whole new era which went far beyond Pont-Saint-Esprit to the rest of the world. No one could tell where it might end.

The evidence was stronger now than it had ever been. Ergotism, especially in the light of the traces of ergot found in the analyses at the Marseille laboratories, was unquestionably the probable cause of the rare outbreak. The last stumbling block had been overcome, theoretically at least: How to explain the manner in which such minute quantities of ergot could carry enough concentration to create such lethal results.

While the evidence was overwhelming, there was still no positive proof in hand. The facilities in Switzerland were actually the only place that the subtleties of the new drug and all its implications could be studied. The police laboratories knew practically nothing about the new drug, to say nothing about how to analyze it. No other toxicological laboratory at that time could report intelligently on the new form of lysergic acid which still mystified even its creators.

The doctors knew that they could not release any irresponsible or hasty information on the new development. The public, the authorities, the police, could hardly be expected to grasp the significance of an accidental form of a new, mysterious drug without careful briefing. The social implications of the drug beyond the local scene were staggering, yet how could the layman grasp it in its full light?

Dr. Giraud and Dr. Latour, after the meeting had been adjourned, and after Hofmann and Stoll themselves went on to Pont-Saint-Esprit to examine the victims, prepared a supplementary report for l'Académie Nationale de Médecine. The paper examined and delineated in detail the similarities between the Pont-Saint-Esprit cases, historical ergotism, and the psychogenic symptoms of LSD-25. They made their findings available to the toxicologists, the police, and the *juge d'instruction*, and went on with their work trying to rchabilitate the *malades*.

The *juge d'instruction*, M. Perrier, failed to show any response to the carefully documented reports, and neither did the toxicologists. Their interest was diverted by a letter received from a Swedish doctor who claimed that he had encountered some cases in Sweden in which his patients had suffered from some of the symptoms encountered at Pont-Saint-Esprit, and that the cause had been traced to poisoning by an organic alkyl-mercury compound used in an agricultural fungicide under the trade name of Panogen. And while long-distance diagnosis is hardly effective methodology, the judge and Commissioner Sigaud seized on this as at least something more tangible and concrete than a strange, new discovery whose properties sounded as if they belonged to witchcraft and the Dark Ages. The mercury and fungicide theory had been bruited about sporadically over the weeks and months of the inquiry, but was not given much serious attention by the doctors, who found no real relationship whatever in the symptoms, or by professional observers, who said that traces of fungicides and insecticides could be found in *any* agricultural product if they were sought hard enough, but not in quantities that were lethal. Also, had not *ergotisme historique*, raging at a time when mercury compounds were nonexistent, revealed symptoms identical to those of Pont-Saint-Esprit?

One newspaper had been pushing the mercury theory at regular intervals, but it was just as persistently discarded, most emphatically, by the dean of the faculty of medicine at Montpellier, who pointed out the high divergence between the symptoms of mercury poisoning and those of Pont-Saint-Esprit. The same basic question applied to the mercury-poisoning theorists as to those who supported ergotism: How could enough tasteless and colorless mercury poison be concentrated to affect several hundred people so violently, and even kill seven of them?

The police had previously been ready to toss out the ergot theory on the grounds that the quantity was not sufficient to poison so many people. The new discoveries of Hofmann and Stoll, which might possibly explain how a tasteless and colorless poison of immense concentration could bring about the damage, especially in the light of historical ergotism, were dismissed as lacking in concrete proof, and too ephemeral to be believed. LSD-25 at this time had not even reached the stage where it was to be first distributed under the labels: POISON—NOT FOR HUMAN CONSUMPTION—EXPERIMENTAL ANIMAL USE ONLY. It was simply not being distributed at all, the public knew nothing about it, and the police were completely wary and skeptical of the entire idea that such power could be concentrated in such minute amounts.

But the mercury idea was something clear, concrete, firm—a theory that could be seized by the hands and mastered by specific, concrete evidence. The toxicologists, knowing little about ergot and its relationship to LSD, also welcomed the mercury theory because of its clear-cut possibilities for proof positive, in well-charted laboratory waters.

But it took until mid-July in 1952 before they were able to come up with a brief, preliminary telegram on the subject, nearly a full year after the tragedy had struck. It would be many months before the full report would be made. As Professor Ollivier had done before, when he revealed the presence of ergot, the four-man team advised Judge Perrier by telegram of their revised findings under the newly oriented laboratory tests:

TELEGRAM
ARRIVÉE

Mention de service	*Origine*	*N⁰ Expedition*	*Nombre de Mots*	*Date et Heure du depart*
	Marseille	8337	245	10 JU 52 15 *heures* 23

EXPEDITEUR: Laboratoire Interrégional de Police Scientifique de Marseille à Monsieur Perrier, juge d'instruction au Tribunal de Premier Instance—PALAIS DE JUSTICE—NÎMES—Gard

NO⁰ 2029 NOUS AVONS L'HONNEUR DE VOUS FAIRE PART DU RESULTAT DE LA CONFERENCE QUI NOUS A REUNIS A MARSEILLE DU 7 AU 9 JUILLET INCLUS STOP NOUS AVONS DISCUTES LES RESULTATS DE NOS TRAVAUX RESPECTIFS ET NOUS NOUS SOMMES ARRETES A CERTAINS D'ENTRE, EUX QUI ONT REVELES QUE INDISCUTABLEMENT DES PAINS INCRIMINES AINSI QUE DES VISCERES DES VICTIMES EN CAUSE COMPRENNENT UNE SUBSTANCE FONGICIDE DONT L'ABSORPTION ETAIT DE NATURE A EXPLIQUER LES ACCIDENTS SURVENUS A PONT ST ESPRIT STOP PAR FONGICIDE IL FAUT ENTENDRE DES PRODUITS EMPLOYES ACTUELLEMENT SUR UNE GRAND ECHELLE EN AGRICULTURE POUR EMPECHER LE DEVELOPEMENT DES MALADIES CRYPTOGRAMIQUES DES VEGETAUX STOP PARMI CES SUBSTANCES ON DOIT SURTOUT CITER DES COMPOSES TRES TOXIQUES DANS LESQUELS ENTRE UNE CERTAINE PROPORTION DE MERCURE MAIS OU LE MERCURE NE JOUE PAS UN ROLE ESSENTIEL STOP OR LA PRESENCE ICI CONSTATE DANS CES PAINS ET DANS LES DISTILLATES DES VISCERES DE TRACES DE MERCURE SEMBLE DEVOIR ETABLIR QUE LES FONGICIDES DE PONT ST ESPRIT NE SONT AUTRES QUE LES COMPOSES CI-DESSUS MENTIONNES STOP DONC NOS CONFIRMATIONS ACTUELLEMENT TRES AVANCEES PERMETTRAIENT DEJA DE CONCLURE A UNE CONTAMINATION ACCIDENTELLE DESTINE AUX EMPLOIS AGRICOLES STOP

SIGN KOHN-ABREST-OLLIVIER-PELLISSIER-DUMAZERT

10 JUILLET 1952
15 HEURES 23

The toxicologists had the honor, the wire said, of informing the *juge d'instruction* of the results of their recent meeting, at which they discussed the results of their respective work, that certain samples revealed the presence of a fungicide, and that by fungicide they were referring to a commercial product used on a grand scale in agriculture to prevent the development of fungi on vegetable products. Among these substances, the telegram stated, was a certain proportion of mercury, very toxic, but where mercury did not play an essential role. However, the presence of traces of mercury here confirmed in the bread and in the distillates of the viscera indicated that the fungicides of Pont-Saint-Esprit are those that are mentioned above. Therefore, the telegram concludes, the confirmations—already well advanced—permitted them to conclude that the cause was an accidental contamination of one or several sacks impregnated by a fungicide employed in agriculture.

Here at last was what the police and authorities were looking for: A down-to-earth, no-nonsense theory which would wipe away every element of mystery, and would certainly not involve a new drug of which no one had ever heard; a drug with qualities so bizarre that even the scientists who claimed to have discovered it might be looked on with suspicion and distrust.

Were the symptoms of mercury poisoning different from those displayed by the Pont-Saint-Esprit victims? Clearly, yes, but the Swedish doctor consulted had said that the clinical manifestations of an organic alkyl-mercury compound were "very variable in their manifestation and depended on the quantity of the compound introduced into the organism and the duration of time that the absorption involved."

What about the opinion of the entire medical corps—nearly twenty of them—treating the victims, from Pont-Saint-Esprit, to Nîmes, to Montpellier, to Avignon? They apparently had nothing to offer except their analysis of the symptoms, and the suggestion of the new and obscure drug that sounded as if it were something out of a witch's brew.

What about the fact that ergot had been the first discovery in the samples, and was so announced by the toxicologist's own telegram shortly after the accidents? The ergot was reported to be in too feeble quantities to bring about such massive poisoning.

Did not the new LSD, a specific ergot derivative, so powerful that it would dwarf any action by a similar concentration of fungicide, answer that question? Again, who could take any stock in a drug for which such mystical action was claimed?

Were not the symptoms of the victims of Pont-Saint-Esprit mystical enough in themselves? Yes, but there had to be some other answer than a colorless, tasteless drug with power which seemed almost absurd.

If this were true, how could a mercury compound have enough concentration to produce the tragic results? There was no real answer to that, but maybe one would be found.

How could the symptoms of historical ergotism, which were identical with those of Pont-Saint-Esprit, point by point, be explained, since there were no such things as fungicides or mercury compounds in use in those days? That was a question that could not be answered, and today's facts had to be dealt with today.

Why had the toxicologists completely ignored the careful and painstaking studies of the doctors who had treated the patients directly at the bedsides? Because they had now found traces of mercury.

Would this mean that the toxicologists, after nearly a year, had made a complete about-face from their first findings of the presence of ergot? Yes, that was the substance of it.

How could these later tests, at a time when all the samples had deteriorated chemically, be more valid than the tests made at the beginning of the research? That was a difficult question.

If the poisoning were due to a mercury compound, why were the deaths and serious illnesses not caused by the clear, specific, unchallenged and key symptom created by mercury: Kidney damage and destruction? This question could not be answered at this time.

But the police and authorities were satisfied. They ruled out ergotism, including the new drug that might explain ergotism, on one and only one basis: The traces found of the elusive and volatile ergot were alleged to be too small to cause the damage, even though it was documented by established clinical evidence that 95 percent of the traces of lysergic acid would disappear from the body within five minutes after injection, that the lysergic acid nucleus is rapidly degraded by the body, that an injection of 0.5 micrograms (half a millionth of a gram) had caused death in an animal laboratory, that the natural amino acids of ergot were many times more toxic than the synthetics, that ergot alkaloids did not appear in the urine or brain, that they disappeared in the blood and muscles of a guinea pig so fast they often could not be found.

In contrast, mercury, even in nonlethal doses, could be stored in the bones, traces could be found months after consumption, it was always present in the urine, the renal damage was predictable and universal, and its lethal action was, by clinical tests, five thousand times *less* powerful than the new form of lysergic acid.

Again, new battle lines were drawn, this time between the physicians, who could not accept the mercury hypothesis on the basis of their first-hand experience with the patients, and the toxicologists and police, who completely ignored the symptoms and the new drug that might possibly explain them.

There was no question that infinitely small traces of mercury were found in the samples and viscera, just as traces of ergot were found at the beginning. Also, the discovery that two of the sacks among the three hundred and fifty seized at the distribution center at Bagnols-sur-Cèze added fuel to the mercury theory, since each was found to be stained, one as if by a yellow liquid, the other as if by a red liquid. The fact that Panogen, the fungicide mentioned by the Swedish doctor, was red in color fortified the police conviction that here was further exact and concrete evidence that they needed, and from that moment on refused to consider ergot, ergot derivatives, or historical ergotism as factors in the case. There was, however, no way of discerning whether the stained sacks were those that held the flour used by M. Briand, since all the empty sacks of many bakers had been mixed up together at the warehouse in preparation for returning them to the Union Meunière distribution system. Thirty-two of the three hundred and fifty had been put aside by the investigators because they were soiled and stained in one degree or another. Two of the sacks were those marked by the suspect stains. When both stains were tested for the presence of mercury, the results were negative. Further tests were planned, however, to determine whether any fungicidal action was evident.

The competence and ability of the police scientific laboratory to detect, analyze, and examine the new forms of ergot that were only in the early stages of discovery remained a disturbing question. Some of the doctors were convinced that only the Sandoz Company, which was the chief pioneer in ergot research, could handle this specific problem. But the police had all the suspected specimens under strict seal; there was no way whatever to obtain flour, bread, or viscera for examination outside the range of police jurisdiction. Further, it was now almost a year since the disaster, and the chances of discovering anything concerning the volatile and ephemeral ergot were probably out of the question.

But two of the doctors decided that the total disregard and casual dismissal of the symptoms and the possible part played by the little-known and monstrously powerful lysergic acid compound could not remain unchallenged. They determined to make secret arrangements for the Swiss researchers to conduct an independent investigation. They knew that it was a desperate chance, that the time lapse was far too great now, even if they could obtain some samples. But they felt they would be totally remiss in their duty if they did not take that chance, slim as it was.

They found one badly stricken victim who had kept one hundred grams of the bread which had affected him and his wife, two of the most seriously poisoned of the *malades*. He had kept the bread aside because he had hoped to have the specimen analyzed privately, but had never done so. He gave it over to the doctors. The bread was old and dry, but they packed it carefully for shipment. There still remained the necessity of obtaining a wide cross section of flour samples to give the Swiss chemists ample room for experimentation. The doctors turned their attention to this ticklish problem, and were frankly stumped.

They could come to only one conclusion: Robbery. Permission was impossible to obtain from the police; plain, unvarnished burglary was the only answer. Like two criminals they plotted their course. It was deep into the night when they arrived at the Union Meunière distribution center in Bagnols-sur-Cèze. The warehouse was dark and ominous. Stealthily, they crept out of their cars, made their way to the gloomy building. By a method that has to remain secret, they gained entrance to the cavernous room where the sacks of flour, still under official seal, were kept. Using a small flashlight, and some thirty small paper bags, one doctor scooped up the samples, while the other kept an eye out the window for the night patrol of the *gendarmes*. Within a quarter of an hour they had collected twenty-eight bags of several ounces each of the various flours, put them into a small carton, and made their way out of the building. Twice the headlights of a car flashed by, and twice they cowered behind the corner of the building until the danger had passed. They reached their car, drove off at a moderate speed to avoid suspicion. They arrived home safely.

But at this point, they realized that they would have to shift their temporary role from that of burglars to that of smugglers. There was no possible way to get the samples across the Swiss boundary without customs clearance.

By another method, which also has to remain secret, the samples finally arrived at the Swiss laboratories without incident.

Knowing that any presence of ergot would decrease geometrically during the long months of delay, they had little hope of success. Nor did they have any.

After several more weeks of waiting, the Swiss chemists wrote back to say that neither the flour nor bread was toxic to laboratory animals, and they saw no further use of chemical analysis.

"No conclusions can be drawn about the samples," the chemists wrote in their letter, "Experiments made on cats and mice have been of no effect. The bread shows no evidence of having caused any poison."

Even though the results were what they expected, the doctors were disappointed and puzzled. The bread clearly had been one of the most toxic specimens. Yet after so many months, it showed no toxicity whatever. Nor did the flour. If all the toxicological research had been handled in Switzerland from the beginning—well, the answer to that question was academic. Somewhere, somehow, the doctors felt, the inquiry was being stifled and misdirected. But without proof of any kind, their position was unsubstantiated.

The announcement of the results of the research and the new mercury theory added another thump to the endless buffeting that the villagers had been undergoing for long months. Some nodded numbly and shrugged their shoulders. Others laughed at the experts, having lost all their respect for them. Others breathed with relief that the search for the cause was over. Others were curious, wondering what the new announcement would mean.

M. Delacquis, as usual, took his pen in hand, and revealed his feelings, and those of many others, in a letter to the press:

> Four French toxicologists have come to make some sensational revelations: LE PAIN MAUDIT CONTAINS MERCURY.

Is it necessary to avow that their declarations, coming after nearly a year of waiting, leave us skeptical and astonished? This is the least one could be.

In effect, if one reviews the affair from its start, one notices the finding of ergot, ergot always, and ergot alone as the cause. All the theories proposed by the professors, the savants, the engineers, and the journalists have been energetically thrust away by those who today affirm that they have discovered mercury.

On October 27, 1951, in response to those articles in the press blaming mercury-based products for the poisonings, Professor Euziere, of Montpellier, gave a formal opinion: MERCURY IS NOT THE CAUSE OF THE PONT-SAINT-ESPRIT POISONINGS.

On October 15, 1951, M. Le Professeur Ollivier said precisely: Ergot is the base of all the poisonings.

On November 7, 1951, M. Le Juge Perrier, gave this information: THE PROPORTION OF ERGOT IN LE PAIN MAUDIT THAT PROVOKED THE DEATH OF GUINEA PIGS, IS NOTABLY SUPERIOR TO THAT CONTAINED IN THE FLOUR.

At the beginning of 1952, le Professeur Giraud dispatched to L'Academie de Médecine de Paris a voluminous report concluding that the poisonings were caused by ergot.

On April 1, 1952: "The thesis of Professor Ollivier is *ergot de seigle*. The guinea pigs undergoing the tests of the research by Professor Ollivier presented the same symptoms as those who were poisoned at Pont-Saint-Esprit, etc."

Is it necessary to continue with the enumeration of the declarations made during this last few months?

If the bread contained mercury, it is not today, but in August of 1951 that it was necessary to say it. If the analyses have revealed nothing in 1951, by virtue of what scientific miracle do they arrive at the present results? And if mercury had not been researched for over 10 months, it is a grave mistake that has been committed.

Whatever the case may be, we will not easily accept the about-face of the toxicologists. There are many among us who have been poisoned, and suffer still, and we will not admit that our rights be overlooked in silence, even if our obstinacy might be contrary to the wishes of those in high places of authority.

There was no question about it, the rumblings against the slowness of the inquiry and the accusations of a cover-up designated as "*raison d'état*" were increasing. Some felt that the national government was willing to do anything to avoid the responsibility of the gigantic damages that would ensue from the poisonings. Others felt that the O.N.I.C., a direct government agency, was trying to stay off the hook, and would resort to anything to squelch the case. The Union Meunière would certainly be relieved if the case were slowed, and many fingers pointed the monopoly out as the guilty one. Why, people asked, did the mercury theory suddenly come up after months of orientation toward the ergot theory? Would mercury as the cause not take the Union Meunière off the hook? they asked. Although it would not remove the Union from civil action against it, the rumor persisted. Mutterings of "cover-up" were heard everywhere. And the biggest question of all as far as the association of victims was concerned: Why had the famous Paris lawyer not even bothered to answer their letters after he had accepted the case?

Whatever conditions were existing elsewhere, the *police judiciaire* were losing no time in following the scent of the mercury trail. Inspector Rossi, of the Seventeenth Mobile Brigade Régionale in Limoges set out to track down every possible delivery of mercury-based compounds in Maillet's region, in Vienne. His orders included the collection of any toxic mercuric materials discovered, including all information on their origin, the sale of any such products in the *drogueries*, the verification of any use of mercuric products by Bruère's bakery, the tracking down of the numbers of the *wagons* that carried the flour of Maillet southward, and any other evidence on which he could lay his hands. As he tracked through the villages and railway stations of Vienne and Indre, Inspectors Guibert and Solignac paralleled his work in the Midi, combing the localities of Bollène, Orange, Bagnols, and other villages in Vaucluse and Gard.

It was an infinitely complex task. The entire year 1953 dragged by as it was accomplished. Rossi, thumbing through the S.N.C.F. records at the railway station at Chauvigny, verified the number of one suspected *wagon*, K. 308-520, tracing its circuitous route after it had left Poitiers on July 9 with a load of miscellaneous parcels prior to picking up Maillet's flour at Chauvigny. But there were other *wagons*, other railway stations, other millers to check, as well as the presence, or lack, of fungicides and insecticides. His copious note pages included infinite detail:

28 juillet 200 qx destination Saint Hypolyte du Fort, wagon n° 7.466.500
29 juillet 200 qx destination Bagnols-sur-Cèze wagon n° 7.468.86
2 aout 200 qx destination Bagnols-sur-Cèze wagon 7.300.740
3 aout 100 qx destination Remoulins Gard wagon H 7.267.017 (PV N° 49)
Expédition du 27-7 wagon K 7.254.699 etait arrivée de Chateauroux, avec un chargement de detail Expédition du 2-8 wagon K 7.300.740 était arrivée de Nîmes avec un chargement de sacs vides destinés au minotier MIRAULT

A labyrinth of pages like this marked the work of every investigator, endless notations to be sorted, analyzed, appraised.

Rossi's conclusions were that the millers in Maillet's region did not utilize mercury-based products for the control of pests and fungi, principally because lime and other products were cheaper. Whether the millers and the *cultivateurs* were using the product and covering up about it was almost impossible to determine. But the whole tragedy was an impossible event. The more anyone tried to unravel it, the more complex it became.

Inspectors Guibert and Solignac, in the Midi, faced the same problems. They sought, as Rossi had in the north, every bottle and can of mercury product they could find. And there were many varieties: Verisan, Ceresan, Prochim 302, Mercoran, Solusanigran, Granisan, Saprosan, Sanigran, Carisan, Sagpa, Certosan, Francosan, Panogen, S.A.C.F.A., many in both powder and liquid form, some soluble in water, some not; some colored, some not; some shipped in metallic bottles, others in cans or crated *bonbonnes*, the large glass carboys sometimes used for this sort of product.

The chase centered on a water-soluble, volatile product composed of an organo-mercurial compound, of an alkyl-mercury type. It would further have to be, according to the analyses of the stains on the suspected sacks and the traces of mercury found in the laboratory, of red color.

The investigators' notes here were equally complex:

Fongicide A. sec: 1.5 percent de mercure—0.95 percent de silicium en combinaison organique de silicate de methoxyethyl-mercure et d'oxide de fer rouge (colcothar ou rouge d'Angleterrre) —mélange pulverulent insoluble dans l'eau.

Fongicide B, humide: 3.5 percent de mercure—0.6 percent de chlore, en combination de chlorure de methoxyethyl-mercure et de carbonates alcalins. Il présente une coloration bleue azure . . . est livrée en tonelets ou boites cartons avec sac en papier Kraft de double épaisseur, contenant 1 kilo de produit.

Of the entire list of organo-mercurial compounds in the area, none were red in color, but four were ochre, the color of one of the stains on the two suspected sacks. However, none of these were soluble in water, and none of them fluoresced under *la lumière de Wood*—ultraviolet—which was a specific property of the stains discovered on the sacks. The police and the toxicologists were seeking specifically a product which would fill all the requirements of their mercury-oriented researches. It would be liquid, bright red in color, powerful and toxic, fungicide in action, an organo-mercurial compound, the stains of which would fluoresce under ultraviolet.

In contrast, the medical men were convinced that the source was most likely to be a derivative of ergot; of extremely concentrated power; able to produce bizarre and incredibly unique psychic symptoms, as shown in the rare instances of history and in the victims of Pont-Saint-Esprit; so volatile that it would disappear except for small traces before laboratory tests could be effected, which would logically account for the minimum traces found in the samples and the viscera. The only logical answer from this point of view would be the spontaneous, accidental, and natural creation of an ergot-related alkaloid with the principal properties of the newly discovered LSD-25, consumed in a massive and accidental overdose.

The answer to the police and toxicologists' search was Panogen, the only compound that seemed to fill the requirements on which the toxicologists were basing their entire research. It was the fungicide that had been suspected in the Swedish poisonings about which the doctor from there had written, although these poisonings were small in number, resulted in no such dramatic psychic disturbances, created markedly different symptoms from the Pont-

Saint-Esprit cases, and were related only to the chronic handling of the fungicide over an extremely long period of time.

Very little Panogen had been exported from Sweden to France. In March of 1949, 5,010 liters had been shipped to a Paris firm. But none had ever been delivered at any time to the regions involved in the wheat, flour, or bread of the Pont-Saint-Esprit case, to the *départements* of Vienne, Indre, Ardèche, Drome, Vaucluse, or Gard—with one exception. A *bonbonne* of thirty liters had been sent in 1949 to Beaucaire, in Gard, for agricultural experimentation. An investigator for the *police judiciaire* was whisked off to Beaucaire immediately on learning of the possibility of pinning down the source of the poison theorized by the laboratories. The *bonbonne* was found, intact and sealed, and it had never been opened, utilized, or damaged in transit.

Even if it had been, the other investigations of the transportation of the wheat indicated that all the *wagons* destined to Bagnols-sur-Cèze with the flour that arrived in the suspected period were filled exclusively with flour, and no evidence of broken bottles, or mercury products was found.

The final report prepared by the four toxicologists—so long in the making—was voluminous and painstaking. But nowhere in it did they relate the findings of the traces of mercury to the symptoms, or acknowledge the possibility that the new discovery of the lysergic acid derivative had any possible bearing on the case.

"In certain samples of the bread," the police summary of the research states, "the experts have discovered the presence in very feeble quantities of *ergot des céréales*. . . . But these elements have always been found in quantities too feeble to be, according to the experts, the origin of the toxic accidents. The ergot notably, which had been suspected at the beginning, has always been found in quantities inferior to one (1) per thousand.

"It is therefore," the police report concludes, "correct to abandon definitely the first hypothesis envisaged, that of poisoning by ergot."

With this brief statement, the doctors were summarily dismissed and sent to pasture.

The police and the toxicologists made no mention of the fact that the quantity of "one per thousand" was literally a gigantic dose if the poison were akin to LSD-25, of which as little as a quarter of a millionth of an ounce could cause hallucinations that would last for hours. If this tasteless colorless form of lysergic acid could cause such a reaction in this tiny proportion, what could a massive dose of "one per thousand" do? Again no one knew, and no one would make such an experiment on human beings. Unless this had already happened by accident at Pont-Saint-Esprit.

With mercury requiring up to five thousand times as much strength as lysergic acid for a fatal dose, there is no mention in the police reports why the mercury hypothesis was not discarded with the same casual manner as was the lysergic acid theory: on the basis that the quantities of mercury found were too feeble. It is true that the toxicologists found traces of mercury, and that the specimens exhibited fungicidal action when applied to experimental fungus growths. All through the report, filed jointly by the four experts, there is reference to how the samples of bread or flour, as well as the viscera, were able to cause fungicidal action.

But it is here that the toxicologists failed again to mention a critical point, one that could challenge their entire theory. *Some molds contain their own fungicide* and are actually able to kill fungi, just as antitoxins can create immunity. *Griseofulvin,* for instance, is a fungus used to destroy other fungi. *Nystatin* is another. Nowhere did the toxicologists mention this possibility in their report, nor did they seem to emphasize that (1) there was less mercury evident than there was ergot and (2) ergot in the form of a lysergic-acid compound could be many times more powerful than mercury.

In addition to bluntly dismissing the possibility of ergotism, as advanced by the doctors treating the patients, purely on the basis that the quantities were thought to be too minute, the report indicates that all the research was oriented toward the fungicide principle. The findings of "a substance possessing the toxicological identification characteristics of the active principles of ergot, a parasite of grain"—which Professor Ollivier had mentioned in his letter of October 15, 1951, to Judge Perrier—were not considered significant in the new report.

All the tests in the autopsy of M. Mison's dog—from hypnotic barbiturates through alcohol, chloroform, cyanide, phosphorus, arsenic, antimony, and even mercury—were negative. But since the research was oriented toward the fungicide theory, the toxicologists applied special tests on other samples for organo-mercurial traces, and were able to find a trace in the proportion of only 1 to 500,000. They also found a trace of a group of unidentifiable alkaloids, which indeed could have been ergot. The extremely weak presence of the organo-mercury traces was explained as being the result of its volatility. The unidentified alkaloids were not able to be deciphered.

In the case of the viscera of the first three human victims who died, the final opinion arrived at the conclusion that "the toxicological examinations, looked at in ensemble, permitted the conclusion of the presence in the viscera of a complex substance characterized by mercury. . . ." But again, this was in the proportion of 1 to 500,000.

Another alkaloid discovered in the viscera is dismissed by the comment that "it does not possess the particular characteristics of a toxic alkaloid; it is perhaps a *ptomaine banale,* without interest."

The findings of "the characteristics of toxicologic identification of the active principals of ergot, parasite of cereals," which Professor Ollivier had mentioned in his letter of October 15, 1951, to Judge Perrier, were lightly dismissed in the new report of the experts.

In the examination of the viscera of young Joseph Moulin, made at Lyon at the specific request of his sister, who was a pharmacist, the conclusion of the experts was that his death was due to *un syndrome nerveux,* of toxic origin, but that the toxic agent was unable to be identified.

The dog of Mison, when tested at the Marseilles laboratory, did not reveal any presence of mercury whatever.

The samples of flour, however, not only failed to reveal any presence of mercury, but revealed the presence of ergot alkaloids in the quantity of 1 to 1,000, which the toxicologists pronounced as a proportion that would be "inoffensive." Before the discovery of LSD-25, 1 to 1,000 was clearly considered a mild dose of ergot. But if, in one of the rare occasions of history, the ergot of the flour in the bread of Pont-Saint-Esprit had spontaneously and briefly mutated into a form of lysergic acid akin to LSD-25, the victims would have been exposed to a dose many times the effective dose of the drug.

The final report of the experts revealed that there was no presence of mercury in the bread at all. Their explanation here is that "if it has not been formally confirmed that an organo-mercurial fungicide was present, it was extremely probable." They go on to point out that the traces of mercury (at the proportion of 1 to 500,000) were discovered in some of the viscera.

There were two *flûtes*—the long, thin loaves of French bread so common in France—and a morsel seized by the police at the *domaine* of Joseph Moulin, baked by M. Briand at the time of the fatal incident.

These revealed, at a considerable time after the seizure, the absence of volatile poisons, the absence of mineral poisons (including the total absence of mercury), the absence of vegetable and synthetic poisons.

The bread samples were well risen, with the normal number of air cells; the bread was well cooked, the flour for the most part was white, and over-all, its aspect was engaging. Under microscopic examination, it revealed wheat flour, rye flour, some bean flour, some crystallization of the flowers of the wheat plant, and further traces of rye mixed with some sawdust of the conifer family. There was ergot "in feeble quantity." (About 1 to 1,000. There was no explanation why this proportion was less significant than the 1 to 500,000 of mercury.) There was also the presence of parts of insects, of mites, of the hair of rats.

In spite of this, the toxicity, when tested by injection in white mice, was negative. Interesting and critically important was the fact that ergot was found, while mercury or any organo-mercurial compound was not found. Yet it proved able to destroy some species of fungus.

The bread of M. Mison, although it was fatal to both him and his dog showed the absence of volatile poisons, the *absence of mercury*, although ergot *was* present in the 1 to 1,000 proportion. There was, in addition, a group of alkaloids which were unidentifiable. Two adult male guinea pigs injected with this sample showed violent contractions of the muscles of the head, followed by a paralysis of the posterior portion of the body, just as revealed by M. Mison's dog on the tragic day he fed it with the same bread. In a few days they became blind, accompanied by a violent aggressiveness, and they died in spasms after nine days.

Autopsies on the animals showed an intense dehydration in all the tissues, emaciation, general congestion, including the kidney, and important vasoconstriction. Again, even *though there was no evidence of mercury being present, the bread was able to create fungicidal action on some species of fungus.*

Most interesting, and generally overlooked in the mass of data assembled by the tests, was the fact that a sample of the bread baked by M. Jaussent, which had caused the flurry of minor illness just prior to the terrors of *le pain maudit,* was powerful enough to kill two white mice within forty-eight hours of eating it. Again, the presence of an unidentified substance was revealed, presenting the characteristics of alkaloids. The bread had no fungicidal action. This was important because of the fact that here was a lethal sample of bread which had been made outside the realm of M. Briand. Further, Mme. Bonzi had been taken to the hospital at Nîmes with the same symptoms as the other victims, although she had eaten only the bread of M. Jaussent. Two others had had the same experience.

In spite of the sureness and confidence of the report of the experts, which dismissed the ergot theory on the basis that they thought the quantity was insufficient, the report presented an alternate which raises more questions than it answers.

Several of the specimens had shown the power to destroy or retard fungus growth, but was the presence of mercury in only three viscera samples in the proportion of 1 to 500,000 enough to cause such monstrous havoc? Why wasn't there *any evidence whatever* of mercury found in any specimen of the flour or bread or in other viscera? If ergot was considered too feeble at the ratio of 1 to 1,000 (but the new and then-unexplored form of lysergic acid showed that this could be a massively dangerous proportion), how could the much weaker mercury—which failed to appear in any of the bread or flour samples—produce such results? What about the mysterious, unidentified alkaloids discovered? If they were unknown, their power and strength was also unknown. Why were they not explored further? Could they have been the new and deadly form of lysergic acid, or allied to it? Again, what about the correlation of the symptoms to the poison? There remained no convincing reason whatever to believe that a mercury-based compound could produce them. There did remain every reason to believe that ergot—lysergic acid—could.

But the *juge d'instruction* and the *police judiciaire* had to make a decision. They could hardly ignore the advice of their own panel of experts, formed at their request. Further, the toxicologists had done a genuinely painstaking job, based on sound experience and knowledge, even if it had been oriented in only one direction. The affair of *le pain maudit* would have to be settled by the police, so that the case of Maillet and Bruère could be permanently closed, one way or the other. With many questions not only unanswered but embarrassingly open, the decision, right or wrong, was made: Nearly three hundred people had been felled by the accidental soiling, with a fungicide with an organo-mercurial base, of a sack transporting flour.

In reaching the decision, the office of the public prosecutor admitted that, in spite of all the research, they were not able to determine where, or under what conditions, and by whose fault or negligence, the deadly contact had been produced. They also attempted to point the finger of accusation at the compound Panogen, but they officially had to admit that there was no proof that it was at the base of the poisonings at Pont-Saint-Esprit.

The doctors who had treated the sick were outvoted, outshouted, and unconvinced. Yet without access to any definitive samples, and with only the mysteries of new possible developments in the strange netherlands of the ergot alkaloids, it was impossible for them to confirm their ideas. Frustrating was the glaring fact that the mercury theory had been accepted, with the question still wide open as to how such a feeble quantity could have produced such damage.

The ergot theory had been rejected for this reason alone. Yet science was on the threshold of new discoveries in a powerful, unbelievably concentrated drug, which for better or for worse, was about to begin to sweep across the world.

But the victims of the poisonings were only academically interested in the cause of the poisonings. They were vitally absorbed with their lost wages, their lost crops, the time spent by others at their bedsides, the past, present, and future suffering, the danger of relapse. The infinite slowness of the experts, the legal process, the police, and the authorities increased their despair and hopelessness. As M. Moulin put it: "We will all be dead by the time justice is rendered."

THIRTEEN

THERE WERE OTHER questions unanswered by the new mercury hypothesis. The outbreaks at Connaux and Saint-Génies-de-Comolas, and the earlier sicknesses among the clients of M. Jaussent at Pont-Saint-Esprit, while not as severe as those which followed in the trail of *le pain maudit*, were clearly related to the bread, and had brought on some of the minor symptoms that the major victims had suffered. Beyond that, the flour that Maillet had delivered to the village of Tercé, in his own territory, had proved toxic to white mice. None of these incidents would bear any relation to the soiling of a single sack of flour, but would indicate a widespread toxic action of varying and unpredictable intensity.

The fungicidal action discovered in the viscera, flour, and bread samples, however, remained unexplained in the ergot theory. There remained only three possibilities under these conditions: (1) There was a fungicide in the bread, which though not as lethal as concentrated lysergic acid, could be strong enough to maintain its fungicidal action after absorption, (2) the fungicide present in the bread would combine with ergot to increase the power of both, or (3) a lysergic acid compound itself included a fungicide action.

None of these possibilities was sought by the prosecuting magistrate, since they accepted the toxicologists' report as it existed, and prepared to close the case.

Strong protests against the mercury theory arose quickly after it was advanced. M. Chabrolin, director general of the Paris laboratory Société pour la Défense des Cultures, pointed out in a letter to the *commissaire* that the toxicity of M.M.D.D., the active material in Panogen, is weaker than other organo-mercurials used in disinfecting the seeds of wheat, and also weaker than mercuric chloride. He concluded that it was not possible to concede that Panogen was able to pass accidentally into the flour in sufficient quantity to provoke serious illness without being noticed. He stated that the red coloring agent of Panogen would be distributed through the flour and stain it to such a degree that it would have been obvious, and would have rendered the flour totally unusable. He concluded his observations by saying that the symptoms provoked had never been observed by victims of mercury poisoning, including the victims of M.M.D.D., and that "the Panogen hypothesis, which incontestably merits deep study, and for which I have given you all the elements in my possession, does not appear to me worthy of being maintained. All the concrete facts I know tend, in effect, to eliminate it."

Dr. A. Swensson, *médecin chef du Département de Médecine professionnelle* in Stockholm, wrote from Sweden that in the serious cases of alkyl-mercury poisoning, the faculty of speech is lost, but the mind or intelligence itself is not influenced, and that confusion and mental troubles are not observed. Where the eyes are affected, the vision is damaged in a very specific way: The patient is able to see out of the center of his eye, but the peripheral vision is blocked by a *champ à lunette*, without pigmentation. In the case of the victims of Pont-Saint-Esprit, the *central* vision was blocked by a large atrophied zone in the center of the retina, *with* pigmentation—the exact opposite of the mercury eye symptoms.

On the witness stand in a Swedish tribunal requested by the French authorities, a biologist and chemist from the manufacturers of Panogen contended that carefully conducted tests showed that if Panogen spilled out on a sack of flour, it would not distribute itself in a homogeneous fashion, but would collect in a single spot and create an extremely hard crust of brilliant red which would be immediately recognizable to a baker who tried to panify it. Further, in the proportions suggested by the French research, the flour or paste would be obviously and glaringly red, even if the crust were broken up and distributed throughout the flour. In addition, this quantity of the compound would contain so little mercury that it would be unable to provoke toxic symptoms.

Dr. Swensson was also called before the tribunal in Sweden. He was known for his definitive study on alkyl-mercury poisoning covering all known cases in Sweden up to 1952. He examined in detail both the chronic and acute poisonings from alkyl-mercury compounds, and the oral and respiratory forms. With strong, single doses, the symptoms of anxiety or mental troubles never appeared. In severe cases of chronic poisoning, they sometimes appeared just before death. One specialist, who was an instructor in the use of the fungicide, neglected to take the prescribed precautions in handling the material, and after a long period of time, was stricken with the chronic form of the disease. He died without any of the symptoms indicated at Pont-Saint-Esprit.

Dr. Swensson compared the over-all symptoms of Pont-Saint-Esprit with those characteristic of alkyl-mercury poisoning and found practically no parallels, especially the pathologic image of the hallucinations. The cramps, convulsions, and gangrene noted at Pont-Saint-Esprit and in the accounts of historical ergotism were never encountered in the framework of mercury poisoning.

Dr. Karl Lundgren, of the staff of the Carolin Hospital in Sweden, took the stand to confirm Dr. Swensson's statements. After a complete study of the French Academy's report of the Pont-Saint-Esprit outbreak, he could find no similarity between that and the poisonings documented for alkyl-mercury. He indicated that a single absorption of any such compound could not possibly produce the pathological picture that occurred in the little French village.

The *police judiciaire* and the *juge d'instruction* of Nîmes brushed all this aside, along with the conclusions by the other doctors who had filed their report with the French Academy of Medicine. There remained now only the preparation of the *Réquisitoire Définitif* and the separating of the charges against Maillet and Bruère as a causal link to the Pont-Saint-Esprit disaster. While it would take considerable time to prepare the official report, the decision was set, and Maillet and Bruère would be free of everything except the charges of *fraude alimentaire* in Vienne.

The final conclusions of the tribunal for the criminal case were to be:

(1) That Maillet and Bruère were charged with *fraude alimentaire* and infractions of the special legislation concerning grains and flour.

(2) That these misdemeanors were alleged to have been committed in Vienne, were not in a proved causal relationship to the involuntary homicides at Pont-Saint-Esprit, and therefore the tribunal in Nîmes (Gard) lacked jurisdiction to handle the case.

(3) That as far as Pont-Saint-Esprit was concerned, the proof had been made that: (a) the bread alone was the cause of the poisonings; (b) the poison preexisted in the flour, but it did not reveal any exterior warning in odor or color or other signs; (c) the toxic agent was composed of a complex organo-mercurial compound, volatile, of the alkyl-mercury type; (d) the toxic had strong fungicidal action, and showed the properties of a commercial fungicide colored red; (e) a very small number of sacks had been found which had been stained by the fungicide, and they were probably stained by the spilling or breaking of a container of fungicide; (f) the product spilled on at least two sacks (although the sacks were not actually proved to be those which M. Briand used) which were filled and sealed, the liquid soaking through the sack, which in turn was able to absorb most of the coloring agent; and (g) in spite of all the research, the investigation had not revealed "in what condition and by the fault of whose negligence the deadly contact had been produced."

The enfeebled Association for the Defense of the Victims of the Poisoned Bread at Pont-Saint-Esprit followed the proceedings against Maillet and Bruère with continued impatience and despair. While the findings of the criminal case would be the basis for their civil action, they had inexplicably heard nothing more from the Paris attorney, M. de Moro-Giafferri, and finally reached the painful conclusion that they never would. Maître Tailhades was likewise unavailable.

They never found out the reason why de Moro-Giafferri had accepted the case, and over two years later, dropped it without ever talking to the victims or writing them. But they did find one of the most prominent lawyers in Nîmes who would accept the case, an *avocat à la cour d'appel* of high stature and boundless energy.

Handsome, magnetic, and powerful, Maître Charles Bedos was known for his passion for taking on tough cases, his infinite attention to detail, his tenacity, his support of the underdog. He accepted three days before *les fêtes de Noël*—the time in Pont-Saint-Esprit when the cheer of Christmas is mixed with the dubious blessing of the mistral, sweeping down the Rhône Valley with screeching force, whipping up strained nerves and wind-lashed tempers. As an *avocat,* M. Bedos would be pleading the case at the Tribunal. Working with him would be, according to French custom, an *avoué,* who would prepare the case in cooperation with him, but not appear in court. Chosen was Marcel Divol, a tousled, graying lawyer, who knew how to combine his capacity for correlating facts with the warmth and wit so characteristic of the Nîmois citizens.

The civil case would have to be prepared, technically, against M. Briand as the seller of the bread that had brought about the tragedy. Under French law, as in many other countries, the vendor is responsible not only for the damages caused by his own negligence, but for the materials under his care, under a normal contract of sale.

The baker, in selling the bread, automatically established such a contract. He is obligated to guarantee the client against "hidden vices," even if he has inherited them from his distributor. The civil code also distinguishes between the seller of bad faith, and the seller of good faith. M. Briand had already been established as the latter, with all the evidence accumulating to show that he had in no way been aware of the "hidden vices" within the flour, regardless of whether they consisted of ergot, lysergic acid, or a mercury compound. But the civil code did not separate the two as far as damages were concerned. Each was responsible not only for replacement of the merchandise, but for the damages ensuing from the use of the merchandise.

The civil code further provides that proof must be made that there is a direct causal relationship between the sale of the product and the injuries resulting from it. All this must present "*présomptions graves, précises, et concordantes,*" as the civil code reads.

All of these conditions had been firmly established by the criminal investigations and inquiry. Bedos and Divol, however, on surveying the dossiers of the case, knew that a decision against M. Briand alone would amount to little or nothing for the victims. If the Union Meunière could be proved ultimately responsible, the case would be meaningful, and the ultimate liability pinned down to the source instead of the middleman, who facing the problems that had stumped all the experts later, could not possibly know of the hidden vices in the flour. Failing permission from the court to make a direct assault on the bastion of the Union Meunière, the lawyers could bring the case against M. Briand, who in turn could sue the private flour monopoly for the damages he would have to pay. With scores of victims suffering long and complex damages, this sum could be astronomical. Ironically, it was not the custom of the small provincial shops in France to carry insurance, and M. Briand had none. If he lost, his only hope would lie in his ability to collect his subrogation rights against the Union Meunière. As the exclusive distributor of flour in the entire country, it would be assured that both the victims and Briand would be fighting a formidable artillery battery of legal talent.

Whatever the battle lines that were now shaping up in the civil legal field, they would be on extremely marshy grounds. The entire premise of the case was based on a single assumption, which the experts, the police, and the Tribunal had totally accepted at face value. It was the brick at the bottom of the pile, and if it crumbled, everything else would crumble with it, leaving total chaos. It lay in the single phrase that had been the basis for the conclusions of the criminal investigation: Except for a mercury-based, water-soluble fungicide, no other poison was capable of producing the mass poisonings.

In the early 1950's it was understandable that this could be accepted by nonmedical people who were not aware of what was going on in the field of ergot research.

But if the police, the authorities, and the toxicologists had given serious consideration to the report by the doctors who had treated the victims and to the French Academy of Medicine, this question would at least have had to remain open.

The report by the clinical doctors to the French Academy concluded:

The remarkable chemical research and experiments of *l'école Suisse* with Rothlin, Stoll, and Hofmann—discoverers of LSD—are newly posed, and deepen the problem by the analysis of each of the alkaloid extracts of ergot and its derivatives.

It is not excluded that nature is capable, in certain circumstances, of elaborating and endowing ergot with similar substances which are highly toxic, as the Swiss toxicologists obtained in the course of their remarkable research.

It is not excluded that other chemicals can intensify and hasten transformations of this order.

It is not excluded that the toxic derivatives of ergot are very unstable and are destroyed spontaneously in time.

All this calls for new research. We are only posing these questions.

Has the collective poisoning by the bread in Pont-Saint-Esprit of August 16, 1951, reopened the book where the polymorphic history of collective ergotism is inscribed, which was closed by the grand clinicians at the end of the last century, or does it constitute a new event, imputable to another toxic compound?

It is the toxicologists who must tell us.

With the police toxicologists not interested in such brave new worlds (they would fail even to acknowledge the existence of such a possibility in their 336-page report), the civil case would proceed on the basis of official dogma. What this would mean to the victims would be realized only as the Tribunal pondered, the *avocats* pleaded, and the people waited.

M. Delacquis waited because there was literally nothing else he could do, beyond his continual and exhaustive prodding. When the mistral blew in the year 1954, he had been waiting two-and-a-half years for the action that all his efforts had been unable to stimulate. His eyesight was getting worse. The visual acuity in his left eye was unable to be measured because of the enormous central scotoma blotting out his central vision. He could not walk in the semidarkness without losing his balance and falling. Vertigo was with him constantly. He was compelled to remain in bed for days at a time, forcing himself to get up to attend not only his frustrating work load for the association, but his regular work with the cooperative. Two-and-a-half years after the tragedy Emile had recovered, but he was bent almost double as an aftermath of the seizures he had undergone. Remarkably, he had not lost his spirit or his smile. Along with M. Testevin, undergoing the same relapses as M. Delacquis, he worked in the fields and vineyards after two years of transfusions and special diets. La Villette would never return to normal and everyone there knew it. In every room there were ghosts of the terrifying hallucinations, the memories of the yells, the screams, the horror, the stench.

The selection of Maîtres Bedos and Divol was satisfying. They conferred with the association, amassed the data from the victims, the doctors, the hospitals, then rolled up their sleeves and went to work.

But lawyers cannot work without compensation, and the raising of the funds required for a modest honorarium of good faith turned out to be a major job. Requested was twenty thousand *anciens* francs—approximately forty dollars—yet none of the victims alone could put up this much money. In his fine, classic French handwriting, elegantly scrolled, M. Delacquis prepared a table. Of the victims, only nine could spare the money to contribute. M. Delacquis put his own name at the top of the list, with a contribution of twenty-five hundred *anciens* francs, while Messieurs Roux, Chervieux, Carle, Moulin, Armenier, Crebier, Lapis, and Mme. Dezeuzes were able to scrape together equal amounts to launch the attack.

The final conclusions of the experts and the official police decision had not yet been formally prepared and released. Until that time further action would have to be delayed, because all the evidence of the criminal case would be used for the civil case of the victims.

Again, with impatience and frustration, M. Delacquis wrote directly to the Minister of Justice in Paris, pleading with him to intervene in the case, and to bring certainty into the milky cloud that still hung over the facts as 1954 began.

> For us the drama is that two-and-a-half years after the beginning of the affair nothing has been done to point the exact finger of responsibility, nothing has been realized to compensate the victims, and no justice has been rendered.
>
> After twice officially confirming that the poisoning was due to *l'ergot de seigle*, they have announced that the poisoning is due to

> mercury. It was no longer a question of ergot or ergotine. This about-face obliges one to think that a grave error was committed in the beginning, or the experts have been obliged by outside influences to change the thesis. . . .
>
> Having confidence in your authority, as in your humanitarian sentiments, I thank you for whatever aid you can give in bringing to us all the light possible in this tragic affair. . . .

The scores of letters M. Delacquis had written seemed to achieve nothing, even with an attorney from Paris, who had undertaken to accept the case for the defendants. There was no response from the Minister of Justice, increasing his despondency and sense of helplessness. It was as if he were swimming in a sea of glue, for even with the fresh infusion of energy inspired by Maître Bedos and Maître Divol, the case was barely able to tread water without the official decision being clearly stated and published. In one of his blackest moments of despair, he telephoned to Nîmes to the *juge d'instruction* Perrier and pleaded with him for an audience. With considerable reluctance, it was granted.

He cycled down the hill from La Villette on the morning of March 22, 1954. The mistral, howling along the Rhône Valley, made the pumping difficult, especially with his shaky legs and precarious sense of balance. But he deposited his bicycle at the S.N.C.F. station and walked along the rue de la Gare to the bus stop. His continuing vertigo worried him. Only the night before he had returned from a brief holiday in the Haute-Savoie to see some friends. Walking with them, his legs had gone completely out of control, and even with their help he had difficulty getting back to the house. His legs felt as if he were walking through water. Riding in the nine o'clock bus to Nîmes that morning, a "head full of vertigo," as he described it, returned to him, but he determined not to let it block his plea to the judge for action, which had now been so long delayed. He did not relish the journey—almost an hour each way on a bumpy autobus—but his will forced him to do it, just as it had prodded him to take on the responsibilities of the association. If scores of people had suffered as he had, he knew from his own experience what they had gone through, knew that he could not rest until justice had been rendered. He had full hopes that a personal plea to the judge would bring action as none of his letters had. No one, even a jurist or magistrate, could fail to be moved by the direct confrontation of the story, as opposed to the mechanical records in the legal dossiers.

Even in March the city of Nîmes reflects the aura of historical majesty. The Arena, one of the finest preserved from Roman history, sits beside the Palais de Justice, a gaunt reminder of the bloody battles of the gladiators, who entered it with the sure knowledge that if they weren't killed in the next event, it would not be long thereafter. Not far away the columns of the Maison Carrée and the triumphant Gate of Augustus stood as reminders of the impermanence of civilizations, however mighty in their prime.

M. Delacquis walked with uncertainty from the bus stop to the Palais de Justice, a dominating, massive structure in classic Roman tradition, but built in the eighteenth century to house the tribunals of justice. As he climbed up the broad, stone stairway, pausing for breath at intervals, he was impressed by the solemnity of the building, its severe, foreboding atmosphere. Somehow, he felt, he must overcome this, conquer it on the basis of humanity, on the basis of compassion and understanding, for those in desperate need.

The *juge d'instruction*—somber, severe, detached—was waiting for him in the courtroom. The judge greeted him with the barest of civilities. M. Delacquis, his vertigo returning once more, felt his hopes ebbing swiftly. He could detect no kindness or sympathy. There was not much he could say. He pointed out the urgency for a decision, so that the victims could move in concert against those culpable. He told of the many hardship cases among the victims. He heard the judge explain that the case against Maillet and Bruère would have to end with a *non-lieu,* indicating the lack of sufficient evidence to condemn them; that Panogen seemed to be the only explanation as the sole commercial fungicide that seemed to have the characteristics noted by the *expertise*.

It was a fruitless meeting, and ill-founded from the beginning. As a magistrate, the judge could say nothing specific to M. Delacquis, who was certain to become a principal in the civil plea to be brought before the court. The phantom of uncertainty was still hanging over every individual concerned with the case.

The meeting should not have affected M. Delacquis as deeply as it did. But as he left the chambers of the Palais de Justice, he felt that he had lost all hope for all time. He walked by the Arena, along the Boulevard de l'Esplanade, to a little sidewalk café. The Nîmois citizens, typically bouyant and gay, were sitting at the tables, impervious to the mistral, sipping their *pastis* and chattering amiably. M. Delacquis felt detached from them entirely. He found a small table, ordered a *jambon* sandwich and *café filtre*. He would have liked, in fact he felt he needed, a glass of wine. But his illness would not permit it. His vision, blurred by the loss of most of his vision in one eye, made him withdraw further into himself. In spite of his depression, he summoned up the resolve to see the case through to the end, regardless of the setbacks and uncertainties. He took the four o'clock bus back to Pont-Saint-Esprit and fell into the fitful sleep of total exhaustion.

By late April, when the mistral had tamed down to a shallow sough, the spring was beginning to resurrect the luminosity and beauty of the Midi, and M. Delacquis's spiritual replenishment was increasing, in spite of his physical debilitation. Maître Bedos confirmed to him that the criminal case was all but settled and that the police laboratory experts had filed their final, if not clearly supportable, conclusions. Further, although the decision would place Maillet and Bruère "outside of cause," and remove M. Briand from any criminal charges, the technical civil case against him and the Union Meunière could proceed.

But by July no official word had been issued by the magistrate, and the association of the victims, strained by debt and continued illness, linked their weak hands together. Over thirty of them petitioned directly to the Premier for action which had been so long promised and so slow in forthcoming:

> The victims of *le pain maudit* of 1951, at a meeting on June 28, 1954 . . .
>
> Declaring that 34 months after the beginning of the affair, nothing positive has been issued by the *cours d'instruction*, and that in spite of the enterprising measures and information furnished by the court . . .
>
> Declaring that three months after the submission by the experts of a report on the nature of the toxic to the *Procureur de la République*, no official publication has been made, and the *juge d'instruction* has not yet set forth his conclusions,

Protest one time more against the slowness of the investigation . . .

The petition was sent to the Minister of Justice as well as the Premier, the highest office in France, with a letter from M. Delacquis:

We have hesitated before addressing you this request, the magnitude of the task that you have undertaken being of the nature to demand all your attention and all your time. However, since it is no longer possible for us to maintain our confidence in the regional powers, we have finally decided to write you directly.

The affair of Pont-Saint-Esprit has had a reverberation throughout the entire world, and it would have been good for the prestige of our country for the inquiry to have been made regularly and exempt from all equivocation.

But, nearly three years have passed since the poisonings, and nothing has been truly accomplished, either to indemnify the victims, some of whom are the dead we mourn, or to bring the real truth to light.

The impression among all the victims is identical: The case is intentionally being stifled. For nearly three months, the *juge d'instruction* has recognized that the criminal case can come to no other conclusion that a *non-lieu,* but this has not been announced. Since the final decision was made this long ago, and since the toxicologists have delivered their report three months ago also, we cannot tolerate the comedy continuing any longer. We ask nothing more than for the *juge d'instruction* to order the closing of the criminal case, providing us with the right to act in the civil case.

With my excuses for the disturbance I have permitted myself to cause you, and counting on your humanitarian sense to hasten this matter with all possible dispatch, I pray you to accept my respectful salutations. . . .

At the close of July, 1954, the Premier answered M. Delacquis directly:

By your letter of July 7, you have wished to call my attention to the slowness of the investigation concerning the affair of the poisoning by the bread of Pont-Saint-Esprit.

I have the honor of informing you that in response to the desire that you have expressed to me, I have placed your request in the hands of the *Ministre de Justice.* . . .

Since a copy of the letter had already gone to the Minister of Justice, there was no real progress made in the appeal to the Premier. But M. Delacquis took hope in the fact that the double impact might have some effect in speeding up the case.

In the meanwhile, the association began assembling all the final details of the dossiers of the victims, bringing them up to date with current medical certification. In a new meeting M. Bedos patiently explained to the group the difference between the civil and criminal cases, how the action would be brought against M. Briand, who in turn would bring action against the Union Meunière to assume the amounts of the damages that he would be required to pay if the case were won by the members of the association. He explained that actually it would be a matter of over fifty individual lawsuits—since that was the number of victims who ultimately decided to carry the suit through—proceeding as a group, which in turn would keep the legal expense down for each of the victims. He further explained that one clear and well-documented case would probably be processed as a precedent, so that a precedent could be specific and easily established. The remainder of the cases would then be settled according to the dossiers of each individual. He emphasized that a civil victory for damages against M. Briand would mean little or nothing for the victims, that he hoped the court would allow a joint action so that M. Briand's appeal against the Union Meunière could be decided at the same time. He explained how M. Divol, as the *avoué*, would prepare much of the material for the case, and that he, in turn, would plead the case before the court, as *avocat*.

He explained, above all, that the process was long and painstaking, that the victims must have patience beyond all endurance, even beyond that which they had endured over the three long years they had already waited. He told them about how the Union Meunière had formidable legal talent on its side; how it would use every possible delaying action; how it would undoubtedly appeal any decision made against it. This, he said, must be faced as a fact. In the meantime he would do all in his power to expedite the case, and had great confidence of winning the decision, regardless how many legal complexities they might encounter.

It was a sober, realistic meeting, held in the impressive offices of M. Bedos on the avenue Feuchères in Nîmes, a broad and elegant avenue steeped in Nîmois tradition and reminiscent of Paris in a golden age. The victims, more used to the narrow confines of the Grande Rue, felt somewhat ill at ease. But they were impressed by the stature and confidence of M. Bedos, and they returned to Pont-Saint-Esprit in the rattling bus with a mixture of hope and some apprehension of the continuous waiting and the complexities of the forthcoming legal struggle.

The official report of the decision of the *juge d'instruction* was finally released on August 10, 1954, with the minimum of fanfare and to the surprise of no one. It appeared less than a week away from the third anniversary of the outbreak. It confirmed the acceptance of the mercury poisoning theory, as everyone by this time expected; it made no mention of the conclusions of the physicians who had found no meaningful relationship between the symptoms of the victims and those of mercury poisoning, and who felt that dramatic new discoveries in ergot and its derivatives were being totally ignored.

As the third anniversary of the Day of St. Anthony's Fire approached, M. Delacquis tried to summarize his feelings in a letter to the press. Gentle and sensitive, he was paradoxically a stubborn and relentless in-fighter. Once he had assumed a responsibility, it became almost an obsession with him. He seldom used the word hate, and seldom felt it. Those who knew him best said that the only thing he hated was injustice, that he poured all the venom he had into this, and that was why he had none elsewhere.

On August 12, 1954, his letter appeared in several papers of the Midi:

> In several days, we will be able to celebrate the third anniversary of the tragedy of which we have been the involuntary heroes. . . .
>
> We will not have to organize a parade or a procession, we will not have to prepare, read, or listen to patriotic and fervent speeches, we will not have to praise ourselves again, glass or fork in hand, with self-congratulations for high warlike deeds.
>
> We are more discreet, doubtless more sincere as well. Some words of affectation will rise from our hearts to our lips (or toward our pen holders) to express the infinite gratitude, which soothes our sadness, to all those who helped, soothed, and defended us.
>
> Making honorable amends, we will revise the hasty judgment that we had formulated about the competence of the toxicologists.

We will give thanks to Heaven for having preserved us from premature reports by experts who do not fear when it is necessary to abandon one proposition for another, even if this constraint gives rise in their hearts to a Corneillian drama.

We will not forget, in the fervent homage that springs from our hearts, the Public Powers, the politicians, all the men in a word who gave proof to us of humanity and social sense. Thanks to them, to the speed with which less than one year after the outbreak of the poisoning, the aid has been generous, integrally distributed and without haggling and without shabbiness, the families of the dead and the sick have really felt that they were not abandoned.

Thus, between August 13 and 18 each of us will begin the third anniversary of the poisoning of the bread. All the victims will not share my opinion, but all at least will rediscover that we have had the luck to be well protected. We are thankful that this painful affair has not dragged on in length and resulted in a veritable scandal.

A poisoned one,
M. Delacquis

M. Delacquis's bitterness was understandable, not only because of the three long years of attrition, but because his eyesight was becoming progressively worse, his voice becoming weaker as the physiological aftereffects settled in his throat, and the vertigo confronting him with totally unpredictable problems in keeping his balance.

But in spite of their acceptance of the inconclusive evidence and their rejection of the symptomatic and new research facts being uncovered for the first time, the *police judiciarie* and the *juge d'instruction* were wrestling with one of the most complex cases of toxicology in history, as were the experts on the toxicological panel. The public authorities were equally confounded. M. Delacquis's pleas were for action, and it never came. Many felt that in the light of the complexities of the case the state should have provided more emergency relief on the basis of a natural disaster. Others felt that the Union Meunière should have taken direct humanitarian action voluntarily, if only as a gesture of good public relations, on the basis that they had supplied the incriminated flour. It could, in turn, reserve all its legal rights without prejudice. But the public relations of the organization, as displayed by the tastelessness of the speeches made at the banquet in Poitiers, would hardly give evidence of this type of forethought.

With the way now opened for civil legal action, the association faced again the problem of dredging up more money for the vastly increased costs of the active process. M. Delacquis, in a constant vise between the emotionally charged pressures of the victims and the ponderous machinery of the law, called a meeting just before the cheerless Christmas of 1954 to see where funds could be scraped up from the farmers, the vine tenders, the laborers, and the shopkeepers who made up the bulk of the association.

For the most part, the members were not only penniless, exhausted and racked with lingering sickness; they were in debt. Their faces were almost like the faces of those who have spent long years in prison, with a waxy pallor that no medicine could relieve. Raising money among themselves was as futile as trying to squeeze a certified check out of a turnip. The few who had any spare funds had already contributed to the association to the fullest extent possible.

The decision was made at the meeting to appeal to the town itself for funds to subsidize their legal struggle, which could not actually be placed before the courts until the official criminal investigation was pronounced closed. M. Delacquis wrote the mayor and town council of the village:

> As you are aware, we are preparing to introduce a suit before the civil court of Uzès, with the objective of asking just reparations from all those responsible for damages caused by the affair.
>
> As you also know, the majority of the victims belong to the laboring class and have no funds available for the cost of the procedure.
>
> That is why all the members present have signed a petition that they have charged me to present to you. As their representative, I have the honor of asking you to study their request with the utmost benevolence.
>
> The cost of the legal trial will be approximately 100,000 francs, and we beg you . . . to grant us all or part of this sum, under the form of a subsidy that would be reimbursed after the trial is completed. . . .

The mayor immediately replied that he would bring up the request before the Municipal Council, which was to meet a few days after Christmas in the Hôtel de Ville.

They met, and voted unanimously to approve the grant as part of the village budget, necessarily subject to the approval of the prefect in Nîmes.

Within a month, they received a reply:

> Préfet du Gard — RÉPUBLIQUE FRANCAISE
> 2eme Division — Nîmes le 24 Janvier 1955
> 3eme Bureau — LE PREFET DU GARD
>
> à Monsieur le Maire de Pont-Saint-Esprit
>
> OBJET: Budget Communal—Attribution d'une subvention
>
> You have submitted to me recently a deliberation of the Twenty-ninth of December by which the Municipal Council of your commune has submitted a favorable opinion for the request for a subsidy of 100,000 francs, presented by the "Association for the Defense of the Victims of the Poisonings of Pont-Saint-Esprit," and have moved to include this payment in the communal budget.
>
> I have the honor to inform you that this deliberation cannot receive my approval.
>
> LE PREFET

By now the series of false hopes, quickly shattered by counteraction of some kind, had come to characterize the pattern of nearly every move the association attempted to take. The pattern was joked about at first, but when it became so persistent the members experienced a wide spectrum of feelings, from despair to resignation, to anger, to bitterness, to a sense of apathy. Some felt that the luck would have to turn, that all the setbacks in the pretrial period would foreshadow greater success as the case came to a head. Certainly, they felt, the raising of false hopes would at least fade, and the disappointments that followed them would be correspondingly less.

M. Delacquis, bitter with disappointment about the lack of support for the legal action, regrouped his forces and began pulling together whatever funds and information he could to move toward the ultimate civil trial.

Each victim who could borrow the 2500 old francs, plus 150

francs in stamps, was asked to do so. The members who had some reserves of their own lent the money, or helped the poor borrow it. The major cases were given special attention in the hope that the minor cases would fall in line if the major pleas were won. A total of forty-five dossiers were assembled by M. Delacquis, including social security numbers, specific medical certificates, records of lost income, medical expenses, home nursing assistance, and receipts for whatever cash contribution was made for the legal expense.

Within the confines of the evidence accepted by the police in the criminal investigation, the case of the first victim to die, M. Mison, emerged as the logical one to act as a pilot case. His autopsy had been the only one to reveal a faint trace of mercury, if that were the accepted cause as outlined by the police toxicologists. In addition, the Widow Mison had suffered severe setbacks as the result of her own poisoning. At the age of sixty-eight now, she had had to close their farm shortly after the tragedy and was living with friends at some distance from Pont-Saint-Esprit. Her need for funds was one of the most acute. She had, however, some savings, which along with her small widow's pension, enabled her to avoid becoming a state dependent.

The uncertainty in regard to the source of the poison hung over all the preparations for the trial. The criminal investigation of the police had, by elimination, seemed to settle on Panogen as the source of the poisoning, in spite of the doctors' ergot theory, in spite of the testimony from Sweden, and in spite of the fact that no Panogen had been delivered or found either in the area of Maillet and Bruère or in the region of Pont-Saint-Esprit. The one exception was the carboy that was sealed and had never been opened by the experimental laboratory that had obtained it. The source of the poisoning remained another phantom hanging over the case, elusive and ephemeral, challenging the ingenuity of the lawyers as they thumbed through the voluminous dossiers delivered to them by M. Delacquis.

The detail work in assembling them was back-breaking. It involved correspondence with doctors, employers, welfare clerks, hospitals, relatives—all without the use of the phone except in rare cases. Practically none of the victims could afford a phone, and the association itself had no money in its budget for such a luxury. On rare occasions M. Delacquis would use his office phone, but only before carefully recording the call and paying for it out of his own pocket.

All through the spring of 1955 M. Delacquis worked under extreme pressure, hoping that the loose ends and revised information for each of the dossiers could be completed in time to launch the trial before summer. Delacquis, Bedos, and Divol insisted on verifying facts and eliminating exaggerated or deceptive claims that could seriously damage the success of the trial, and this slowed down the work. When July, 1955, finally arrived, it was obvious that no court action could be scheduled until at least the fall, and M. Bedos wrote to M. Delacquis:

> In answer to your letter of July 4, I must say that I share in your long series of disappointments. However, it is too late to begin the proper procedure, since the judiciary vacation period begins on July 13, 1955. We will be able to proceed again at the end of the vacation period, which is September 10, 1955. . . .

If the legal machinery stopped for the summer, M. Delacquis did not. He continued to make long lists of the materials still missing from the dossiers, attempted to explain to each victim the necessity for precision in filing the cases, counseled, comforted, and pacified. But September arrived, and still no date had been set for the trial.

Meanwhile, tragedies happened, totally unrelated to *le pain maudit* itself. One member was electrocuted while working, and his case was transferred to his wife, as successor. Others lost heart and dropped out of the association. One widow wrote M. Delacquis that she had moved her small son away from Pont-Saint-Esprit because he could stand it no longer:

> I would say that I have made a great sacrifice in leaving my house and all that is dear to me. But I do this for the health of my little boy, who was so badly stricken by the bread, and who spent so long a time locked in the hospital. But now, at least, he no longer hears his friends say to him: "Since you ate the bread, you are crazy!" Let us hope that our patience will serve us well, regardless of how deplorable everything is at the moment.

M. Delacquis wrote her, inspiring her with courage, and indicated to her that by the beginning of the new year 1956 he was confident that the Civil Tribunal at Uzès would be ready to begin the process.

It was now October, the dossiers were complete, the request for the trial had been filed in Uzès, a neighboring city to Nîmes. Hopes were beginning to rise.

M. Delacquis had never been involved in a legal process of this sort. As 1956—the fifth year after the tragedy—was ushered in, he felt, along with the others whose hopes were rising, that the results of all their labor would be fulfilled, that the suffering of all those who had been stricken would be reasonably reduced, and that they could return to a normal path of living in the charm of the little historic village on the Rhône.

FOURTEEN

THE INQUIRIES of the members concerning the progress of the case were for the most part timid, soft, and apologetic, but they were persistent and voluminous. M. Delacquis parried them as best he could, hoping always to be able to make a definitive announcement of the date of the trial. The parade of callers at his office and La Villette tried his patience mostly because of the frustration of being able to do nothing constructive about hastening the process. There were also the letters from those who had to leave town as a result of their illnesses, especially Mme. Mison, whose case was to set the precedent for the rest.

After four more months of waiting, and concerned about the burden she was imposing on her friends by living with them as a semi-invalid, she wrote again asking for any further news.

M. Delacquis, fearing now to give any reply on the delays, which were beyond his control, forwarded her letter to M. Bedos, who was having his own problems with the slowness of the process. The transfer of key criminal dossiers from Marseilles and Poitiers had imposed long waiting, in spite of his efforts to expedite the action. His frustration, too, was increasing as he opened the letter of April 14, 1956, from M. Delacquis, four months after all had thought the trial would be in action:

> The many requests for information on the progress of our case continue. I have given as many explanations as I can, but I think you understand that the members seem to feel that it is drawing out longer and longer, without casting any doubt on your good faith or mine. In this regard, I am enclosing the letter I have received from Mme. Mison, along with my reply to her begging her to have patience. I hope sincerely we will be able to calm very soon the alarm that so many of the members of the Association have expressed. . . .

But the delays continued.

The Union Meunière, whose liabilities were to be assessed in the same court action, benefited by delay after delay. The entire year 1956 went by without a date for the trial being set. But at last the date of May 23, 1957, was announced. The flour monopoly immediately asked for further postponement.

After a full year had gone by, making the total six years since the tragedy itself, even the professional patience of Maître Bedos snapped. In writing the President of the Tribunal at Uzès on May 16, 1957, he said:

> I have come to learn that [the attorneys for the Union Meunière] have asked for a delay of this matter. . . .
>
> Without losing any more time, I have the duty to inform you that, in the name of some fifty clients who have placed their confidence in me, I regret I must personally oppose this new request.
>
> The interests of my clients do not permit them to suffer any new delays.
>
> The damages that they ask for reparations go back to August in 1951, a total of nearly six years. If they were not able to enter their action until 1955, it was because of the long and exhaustive criminal investigation, which lasted over four years.
>
> For eighteen months we have awaited the procedure. If another postponement is granted, it would mean that the process could not begin until after the judiciary vacations—in other words, until next fall. . . .
>
> I have the honor, Monsieur le President, of informing you that

I will present myself at the bar on May 23 to oppose any further postponements. . . .

Receiving a copy of the letter, M. Delacquis was cheered by the strong and resolute stand taken by Maître Bedos. A telephone call to Maître Divol, who was also hard at work on the case, confirmed the fact that any suggestion of a further move for postponement by the lawyers of the Union Meunière would be vigorously opposed. M. Delacquis passed the news along to the other members, who now felt that at last the case was about to break.

At issue was the contention by the monopoly's lawyers that the court at Uzès was not competent to handle the trial, and that the Union Meunière should be removed from the action, leaving M. Briand to stand alone.

It was a ticklish legal problem, technically, with enough doubt cast on the question to enable the flour monopoly to force the court to give it serious consideration. M. Delacquis, fighting for patience, waited for May 23 and the decision.

He learned of it, by letter, from M. Divol on the following day:

> You have been kept abreast of the difficulties arising from our adversaries, who in the last minute have appealed for an additional postponement. At the hearing today this has been granted, moving the trial date until next fall, after the judiciary vacations.
>
> At the audience today the new date has been fixed for Thursday, October 10, 1957, and 9:00 hours.
>
> Your *avocat*, M. Bedos, was present at the hearing when this new date was fixed. . . .

M. Delacquis read the letter with incredulity. By now his reaction to this type of news was almost automatic. He reached for his pen, and quickly composed a letter for the journals:

> For six months, the date of May 23, 1957, has been fixed for the commencement of the legal action by the association of victims against the baker of the bread. It has now been postponed at the request of the Union Meunière.
>
> This organization, having had eighteen months to reflect on its action, has taken a step that is without excuse in our eyes. It waited

until eight days before the trial date to protest that the Tribunal at Uzès did not have jurisdiction.

The victims, who have been waiting for six years to appeal to justice for their legitimate rights, vigorously protest against this maneuver, which is nothing more than an attempt to drown the affair, exhaust our patience. Our protest is academic, we realize, but we trust that public opinion will understand our logic and support us without reserve.

Public opinion or not, the trial was finally set for October 10, 1957. The ancient city of Uzès, the first duchy of France, rises like a fairy tale, turretted sand castle at a point where the Cévennes and the Garrigues roll into each other. Not far away is the stately Pont-du-Gard, the Roman aqueduct that poured gallons of fresh mountain water down to Nîmes. Into this Roman and feudal atmosphere came the lawyers for the Union Meunière—one from Paris, the other from Nîmes—still protesting vigorously that this provincial court had no jurisdiction over such a case. Also arriving were the distinguished and aristocratic Maître Bedos, along with his gruff and witty associate, Maître Divol. The victims came, too, those who could, moving in a caravan along the straight long rows of plane and poplar trees on the road from Pont-Saint-Esprit, tunnels of shade from the Midi sun, which even in October was broiling.

M. Bedos began his eloquent plea at nine fifteen that morning. The three-man panel of judges sat in somber dignity, as he began to review the infinitely complex details of the case. On his plea were riding the hopes of the fifty-four victims who pressed their cases, whose total damages would run into millions of francs. His attack, technically against M. Briand, centered on Article 1641 of the Civil Code, whereby the seller must protect the buyer from "hidden vices," even if he is unaware of those vices. But actually, the guns of the claimants were trained on the Union Meunière, who would, if the action were successful, be forced to relieve M. Briand of the damages he would be required to pay the victims.

For ninety minutes Maître Bedos outlined the individual cases and the legal obligations of both M. Briand, as the defendant, and the Union Meunière, as the third party in the case. He concluded: "The mystery still remains with us in its entirety. But it is not a question for us to judge the lack of final information. We face the fact that scores of victims have been destroyed both physically and financially by this tragedy. These unfortunates, these who have suffered so greatly, these mothers of families who are confined to their beds, these children who must carry their scars the rest of their lives must be indemnified!"

Maître Fontaine, representing M. Briand, pictured his client as a victim of the system that did not permit him to choose his own flour, who had complained in vain about the quality of the flour he was receiving, and who remained a victim himself as a result of the negligence of the Union Meunière.

In turn, the Union Meunière's two lawyers pleaded that their client remained outside of the cause of the poisonings, that it was merely a transporter of a product, that there was evidence that the sacks of flour used did not come through regular channels, that M. Briand, and he alone, was responsible.

For seven long hours the lawyers argued before the court. It was strangely anticlimactic. M. Delacquis listened to the endless technicalities as if he were in some kind of a daydream. It all seemed unreal to him. The end of the road was in sight, after the long years of attrition. There was no sense of elation, even though he was confident that as the facts were unrolled before the court, there could be no doubt that the members of the association would win the case. He felt only a vague sense of relief, that for better or for worse, the struggle was approaching the end.

At the conclusion of the long hours of pleading, he was exhausted. Vertigo had struck him several times during the speeches, times when the chamber of the Palais de Justice spun in a senseless whirl in the middle of endless verbiage. When the last plea was over, he marshaled his nerves, sat forward, waited for the final word from the panel of judges. He knew that an immediate decision would not be forthcoming; that the facts would have to be studied. The *Ministère Public* would have to make his plea of prosecution, and the decision of the court carefully rendered at a later date. He hoped and he felt confident that it would be only a matter of days. After the long attrition he felt he could not face the strain of another protracted period of indecision.

The President of the Tribunal spoke in measured tones as he summarized the straggling and uncombed legal problems. He stated that he would review all the pleas as rendered during the day, but because of the intricate problems involved, the *Ministère Public* would require two more months in order to prepare the public prosecutor's summary. The date for the summary and conclusions would be set at December 12, 1957—a date which would mark six and a half years after the strange malady had swept through the crooked streets of Pont-Saint-Esprit. The decision would then follow at a later date.

M. Delacquis arrived back at La Villette late that October evening. He felt only numbness and apathy. Two months more of waiting seemed to be simply an extension of the pattern he had been following for over half a decade. He collapsed into his bed, where the memories of his vivid hallucinations and the almost-irresistible compulsion to jump out of the window still haunted him. The wheels of justice were not even grinding. They seemed to be stalled.

On the days that followed, M. Delacquis swallowed his anger, which again began to smolder, and tried to put out of his mind the continuous frustrations he was facing. Within two weeks, however, new word was received: Still another postponement was granted.

Instead of a two-month delay before the decision would be rendered, there would be at least a three-month wait, or possibly longer.

With a bitterness that he could not overcome, in spite of his efforts to do so, he dictated a succinct memo to be circulated among the members of the organization:

> For motives of which we are ignorant, the plea for prosecution by *Monsieur le Ministère Public,* which was to be pronounced before the Civil Tribunal of Uzès on December 12, has been remitted to a later date, possibly January 8, 1958.
>
> That is all that the secretary of the association is able to say at this time, keeping provisionally for himself the reflections that suggest to him the incoherence and evasions in an affair which has endured for six and a half years.

The new date was actually set for January 9. In the French system of law the *Ministère Public* launches an opinionated attack, even in civil cases. He assesses the pleas of both claimant and defendant, then presents his conclusions before the panel of judges. While the final decision is rendered by the judges, the *Ministère Public* arrives at his independently, and presents his conclusions very often with passion and eloquence.

While again no immediate decision would be reached on January 9, at least the association of victims would learn the assessment of the merits of the case by a public official.

M. Palavesin, the *substitut du procureur de la République,* served as *Ministère Public* at the audience which reassembled in Uzès on January 9, 1958.

The cause of the victims could not have been served better. Speaking with impassioned conviction, he addressed the court:

"Life is delighted at times to create those reconciliations which are not surprising.

"These vaulted halls in this ancient duchy of France, where die the echoes of a prestigious past, offer you, Messieurs, Judges of Uzès, the distinction and formidable privilege of making the voice of Justice heard in an affair that seems predestined for these rooms.

"In the twentieth century, in the Atomic Age, at a moment on the threshold of the absolute Reign of Science, you must give your judgment as magistrates and as men in a process which touches on that which we hold most precious, the lives of our fellow men, in a trial where even Science has stammered, and through its most eminent representatives, has evoked in us the historical image of this mysterious plague and hallucinatory ghost of the Middle Ages, *le mal des ardents.*

"It is most wrong that one believes that the only predatory criminal is that of Emotion . . .

"Six years after the horrible nightmare of that night in August of 1951, and of the following days, I am, like yourselves, deeply moved and upset to the depth of my being by these deaths, these demented souls, these disabled, these *malades,* these horrifying sufferings, physical and mental, which demand today that we search out and find for them a humane solution in the process of our Law.

"It would be despairing—and the idea of Justice would not even exist any longer—if our process of law did not compensate the injured for their profoundly legitimate interests.

"More than ever I feel the formidable honor of exercising the duties of the *Ministère Public,* this very French institution which, since Montesquieu and Portalis, 'must give through the organ of the Law, a consoling force to the oppressed and the feeble, an accusation against the culpable, a safeguard to the general interest, and a representation for the entire body of Society.'

"Let me swear to you that if my duty is thus clearly defined, I measure also the limits of my own weakness.

"You are, *Messieurs les avocats,* the auxiliaries of our formidable justice by your talent and your culture.

"I have in my memory, as a piercing echo, the harmony of words and pleadings that during long hours have fascinated us . . . and I have also found in the voluminous dossiers the substance of subtle dialectics.

"All this has been impressive, and the man feels discouraged, and the judge begins to doubt himself . . .

"Is it truly so difficult, or even impossible, according to the thesis of the Union Meunière, to give satisfaction to those citizens who are so right in claiming Justice?

"I refuse to believe it!

"The sole and legitimate interests of the victims of Pont-Saint-Esprit will be my only care, and I think it will be done only with the care of Truth and Justice, which is yours to grant.

"My case, which I would like to be brief and clear, will be to follow as objectively as possible the theses of the different parties . . . and to propose to you a solution, a solution which is based on irrefutable facts, and which finds its justification in our law."

He continued, with equal elegance, to analyze the case. Three parties were involved, he said: The victims, the baker, and the Union Meunière. He reemphasized how the baker is held under an obligation to guarantee his product against hidden vices, whether he acted in good or bad faith. There was no question that M. Briand acted in good faith, but if a "chain of causality" could be established between the bread and the poisonings, he would still be responsible.

And there was no doubt remaining, he added. "I have read the report of the criminal investigation, Messieurs, with the greatest attention," he said, "and often with my heart strained with emotion. Permit me to say that this chain of causality is doubly proved within it. . . . I measure my terms when I say to you that this dossier will furnish you without discussion the elements of proof that you need for your decision."

He indicated his surprise that the Union Meunière had not been named as a direct defendant, but only as a third party to whom M. Briand could turn in order to relieve the damages he would be required to pay. "A process earned against M. Briand," he said, "will represent nothing for the victims. I will go further: Such a result in practicality would create another victim, and the list is already too long."

"I will pass to the baker Briand, and I will be very brief," he continued. "This unfortunate man, who has been smothered on all sides by all the transgressions of Israel . . . has called into cause the Union Meunière, supplier of the flour, which he has been forced to utilize. In the second part of my conclusions, I will make—without passion—the defense of this artisan who has nothing for which to reproach himself."

Then, with a dramatic pause, the *Ministère Public* continued: "I come at last to the Union Meunière.

"It is with the greatest of interest that I listened to their two eminent lawyers. I am pleased to praise, in his absence, the young and vigorous talent of M. Chaumie, who had come down especially from Paris."

He paused again, perhaps with the intent of stimulating any disdain the panel of judges might have for an expert from out of town, who had been among the most vociferous in insisting that the little former duchy of Uzès was no place for an important trial like this one.

"Two lawyers," he continued, "two voluminous dossiers, gross quantities of law and fact. . . . All of this was at first impressive. But this accumulation, this superabundance of offensive and defensive material has rapidly led me to think that this famous bastion, the Union Meunière, remaining aloof from the direct demands of the victims, insufficiently attacked by M. Briand, had nevertheless foreseen and appreciated the just value of the danger which certainly ought to weigh on it. . . ."

The lawyers of the Union Meunière, already smarting under the attacks of Messieurs Bedos and Divol, now found themselves facing an even more ferocious attack than before.

As the *Ministère Public* continued, M. Delacquis's hopes rose further than he had ever allowed them to rise. Here was a servant of the state, backing up the attacks that had been prepared and launched by the victims' own lawyers, and doing so with almost irresistable passion and conviction.

The *Ministère Public* summarized the defenses of the Union Meunière as falling into three contentions. "First," he told the court, "they have refused combat before your jurisdiction. They would prefer another terrain of their own choice, which would give them more time to try the patience of the victims who plead against them. . . ."

He pointed out how the Union Meunière would like to picture itself as an arm of the state, that it was strictly dependent on it and under its control. "Better yet, and this gambit is rather subtle, this Union Meunière presents itself as if it were the god Janus. As such, it pretends to play a very modest role, an insignificant role, not carrying with it any responsibilities. As such, it rebukes itself, and taking refuge with a false modesty . . . in the bosom of the state. . . ."

"Second," he continued, "the Union Meunière tries to play another game, which it handles as a magician would. It brandishes its traps in the face of an adversary already blinded. . . ."

He explained how the Union Meunière claimed that its relationship with Briand was a contractual one, which would alleviate many of its responsibilities.

Third, the *Ministère Public* indicated, the flour monopoly had pleaded that proof was lacking on the identity of the polluted sacks of flour. "If we are to believe the Union Meunière," he said, "it would emerge from this trial whiter than the flour it delivers. . . ."

He then summarized three basic contentions—that it was proper for the baker to carry an action against the Union Meunière, that the Tribunal was competent to judge the case, and that the case must inevitably end with the condemnation of the Union Meunière.

As the *Ministère Public* began his long and painstaking analysis of the legal technicalities, M. Delacquis gained more fresh confidence that the fruits of his long struggle were certain now to ripen and endure. The *Ministère Public* pointed out how the monopoly was indisputably required to investigate immediately and take samples of any complaints of inferior flour, how it had ignored all the protests of all the bakers in the area before the tragedy of *le pain maudit* struck Pont-Saint-Esprit. He showed how the organization acted for profit, as a private monopoly, and was not merely an agent of transport for the flour.

He emphasized that the Union Meunière had two uncontestable duties—the duty of general prudence; and the duty of special obligations under its contract, which included the care of the sacks in which the flour was transported and the care of the quality of the flour itself.

"It is of little import," he told the court, "whatever is the exact nature of the toxic agent, whether it is organo-mercurial, arsenic, or whatever—the result would have been the same."

Reaching a climax in his conclusions, he dwelled at length on the condition of the flour itself. "I am coming to the point which is principal and crucial," he said. "I do not wish to exaggerate, and again I measure my terms. This poisoning, hallucinatory, dramatic collective was *bound* to happen; it was bound to happen, having been, so to speak, foreshadowed, foreseen, and denounced in advance.

"It was bound to happen by the fault of the Union Meunière, voluntarily, obstinately passive, in spite of an impressive series of complaints and protests, of pleas brought to its attention in plenty of time to prevent the tragedy."

He paused again for effect, then went on: "What would you think, Messieurs, as well as Judges, of men in the public service of hygiene or health, who received many complaints from a mayor and from citizens in a locality where the drinking water was polluted, and failed to intervene?

"What took place in this case? Among some—with strong bodies, nothing. Among others, an indisposition light and quickly passing. Among others, a malign fever bringing death in its wake!

"This is what happened to the unfortunate inhabitants at Pont-Saint-Esprit. This is the case against the Union Meunière.

"I return again to the report of the criminal investigation, and you will see that the Union Meunière's position is insupportable, and that what we will discover is indelibly inscribed on the physical and moral sufferings of the unfortunate victims.

"These sufferings are simply recorded in the criminal dossier, in the death notices, and in the administrative papers of internment in the insane asylums of Avignon, Nîmes, and Montpellier—the thing that is most poignant.

"What, therefore, were the *boulangers* depending on M. Bousquet in Bagnols-sur-Cèze, and representing the Union Meunière, able to do when they confirmed that the flour was uncontestably bad? They were only able to complain to those who delivered the flour to them. This was their duty. They did it. They all did it.

"But the Union Meunière did nothing.

"To keep this as objective as possible, I am going to let the writings of these bakers in the stricken region speak for themselves . . ."

Then the *Ministère Public* began reading. He read the vociferous complaints of the mayor of Saint-Génies-de-Comolas; the strong and vigorous protests of M. Monier, the baker of Connaux; the deposition of M. Griotti, the other baker of the same town; the protests of M. Bousquet to his own superiors of the Union Meunière, culminating in the urgent SOS sent on August 13—and a similar urgent appeal by M. Bousquet on August 17, one day too late to prevent the tragedy, which was by that time already in action, although no one yet knew it.

"Too late," summarized the *Ministère Public*. "The drama had already begun!

"I have wished to separate these written protests from any commentary that would have been able to dim their light and sinister clarity, preceding, alas the flames of the funeral torches.

"Death spilled out on this land of ours. Our honest artisan bakers, with their good sense, made known their concern and forebodings, and only the Union Meunière remained deaf to this insistent rumbling—a rumbling which foreshadowed, by an implacable logic, the crises of suffering and agony for all the population. Too late!

"The contract between the Union Meunière and the O.N.I.C. clearly states: 'When a utilizer complains about the quality of the flour he receives, the Union Meunière will take at least five samples. . . .' There it is—the last dam holding back the toxic, the only element holding back the eating of the poisoned bread!

"These samples were not to be lifted to confirm the impurities that the naked eye could easily discover, but to see if the flour was wholesome. It was a question of entrusting it to experts, who would utilize a simple experiment on mice and guinea pigs, to discover if it were toxic or even lethal.

"The samples—taken a little after the outbreak—by the *police judiciaire,* have revealed that among one hundred thirteen samples, ninety-nine were totally improper for consumption, and that without searching further. We do not even need to speak of the research reported three years later. Everyone knows that chemicals deteriorate with time. This [later research] signifies nothing.

"The Union Meunière did nothing—and it alone had the power and duty to prevent the catastrophe from happening.

"Consciously, obstinately, it violated its contract, which by its obligations, constituted a dam against the poison, and all other elements unfit to eat.

"Consciously, obstinately, it violated the general obligation of prudence, which is incumbent on every living being in the society.

"Consciously, obstinately, it is guilty of a civil misdemeanor, the cause of all the damage, for which it must answer.

"Voltaire has said that the most beautiful function of humanity is the rendering of justice.

"*Messieurs les Juges d'Uzès,* this honor, for which I envy you, is now reserved for you."

M. Palavesin bowed deeply, moved away from the bench. The courtroom was stilled. The case now was, at long last, in the lap of the Tribunal. M. Delacquis and the Association for the Defense of the Victims of the Bread of Pont-Saint-Esprit could not have had a more moving and eloquent plea.

The lingering and maddening suspicions against the legal process which had haunted M. Delacquis were dissolved. Surely, now, the decision would be promptly made, and the victims for whom he had fought so long would be justly compensated.

By March of 1958, three months after the plea by the *Ministère Public,* nothing had happened.

No sooner had M. Palavesin quoted Voltaire to the bench than the lawyers of the Union Meunière began to assemble their heavy artillery. The Tribunal had permitted them to answer the charges against them by the *Ministère Public,* and now, three months later they did so, in the form of a voluminous tract prepared for them by one of the most eminent jurists in France.

Maître André Rouast was the *professeur honoraire à la Faculté de Droit de Paris,* whose opinion would be tendered respectful attention by any court in France. His opinion could have serious consequences in blocking the only effective action the trial could produce: The ultimate indemnification by the Union Meunière of M. Briand, whose resources would be exhausted before a single case could be indemnified.

His treatise on the case was "a veritable monument of pages," Maître Bedos wrote to M. Delacquis in March, as he explained the new delay that had suddenly arisen.

> Of course, this treatise reflects very lively criticism of the point of view expressed by the *Ministère Public* as far as the Briand-Union Meunière position is concerned. Being given its importance, and although it does not affect directly the position of the association, I believe it is my duty to bring this to your attention. All this will no doubt prolong the deliberation. I do not exclude the hypothesis that the decision will have to be reported only after *des vacances de Paques* [the Easter vacation], but if that happens, it will be once again the fault of the Union Meunière.

In his treatise, the distinguished professor from Paris explored the misty marshlands of the legal intricacies with brilliance and incandescence. He categorically took his scalpel against the position that the Union Meunière was obligated to repair the sins of M. Briand, and cited manifold cases to indicate that the technical questions of law were very questionable indeed. He based his conclusions on two fundamental contentions: (1) The Union Meunière could not be concerned with any negligence action, because the relationship between the organization and the baker was a contractual one. (2) Regardless of this, the Union Meunière would not be responsible because the proof had not been made that it had been guilty of any negligence, and no cause-and-effect had been shown in regard to the poisonings.

The arguments on both sides were centered on the legal problems, not the question of facts. Both sides were forced to accept the report of the criminal investigation as their bible. The conclusions in the report of Professor Rouast were based entirely on the mercury-poisoning theory, which had *not* been accepted by most of the medical doctors as even approximately definitive. The possibility remained open that all the legal reasoning, as tight, expert, and logical as it might be, could merely be creating a well-architected, but highly unstable house of cards. It was a case where the jurists were totally dependent on the opinions of experts and the experts were divided in opinion. Regardless of this, the legal charges and countercharges went on, and the decision of the Tribunal, as surely as predicted by Maître Divol, was postponed again to a date after the Easter holidays.

On April 24, 1958, the judgment was rendered.

For the victims, it was an unequivocal success.

The Widow Mison, highlighted as the clearest case in the line of direct proof, and fulfilling all the requirements of the court, was awarded one million *anciens* francs, a sum roughly equivalent to two thousand dollars. This would have to be paid by M. Briand, but he in turn would be compensated by the Union Meunière, whose arguments to escape involvement failed to move the Tribunal.

All the other victims would have to submit to an appraisal by a board of medical experts, consisting of three members of the faculty of medicine of the University of Montpellier. They would determine the extent of medical damage to each, and the amount of disability reflected by each, verifying that this damage could be traced to the poisoning by the bread of M. Briand.

Only the cases of M. and Mme. Bonzi and one other *malade* were rejected, on the basis that they had not eaten M. Briand's bread, but rather that of M. Jaussent.

In all the cases the Union Meunière was ordered to relieve and guarantee M. Briand for all sums he would have to pay.

Maître Divol, elated with the results, wrote M. Delacquis the day after the judgment was rendered:

> I have the pleasure to forward to you a copy of the disposition of judgment pronounced yesterday in favor of the victims of the bread at Pont-Saint-Esprit.
>
> It is a success. The responsibility of M. Briand is retained, and the denial of jurisdiction brought up by the Union Menuière re-

jected. The appeal in guarantee of Briand is retained. As a consequence, the Union Meunière must guarantee Briand and handle all the condemnations he is required to pay.

We could not have hoped for more.

I am informing M. Bedos of this brilliant result, and am forwarding to him another copy of the judgment.

For the first time in the nearly seven years since his work had begun, M. Delacquis was genuinely proud of his accomplishment. He announced the results of the trial with firm confidence that reparations would begin to be made, and the members would begin to climb their way out of debt.

But the climb that was to begin that spring of 1958 did not even start. The Union Meunière, assigned by the Tribunal to pay the trial costs of seventy thousand francs, refused to pay them, and set about preparing an appeal of the decision of the Uzès court. Since no action could be taken until the title of the judgment was released by the *greffier* of the court, even the sum clearly awarded the Widow Mison could not be sought from M. Briand.

The entire summer passed; autumn was nearly half over when it became obvious that the only way the association could begin any action at all to collect the money from M. Briand for Mme. Mison would be to pay the court costs, and try later to get it back from the Union Meunière. Mme. Mison was now confined to a sanatorium, so weak and ill that she could not leave it. The news of the court decision in April brought her fresh hope that she would be able to repay her friends and relatives who had come to her aid after *le pain maudit* had brought death to her husband and disability to herself.

M. Delacquis, happy to reassure her that direct compensation would soon be forthcoming, found that in November, nearly seven months after the decision, it was impossible to see that she received any money, and with no prediction as to when it might be forthcoming. He wrote her on November 21, 1958:

You have been informed last spring, of the judgment rendered you by the civil court of Uzès.

The *boulanger* Briand has been condemned to reimburse you the sum of one million *anciens* francs in damages and interest, but it is the Union Meunière who is required to pay you this sum.

> M. Divol has informed me that the title to this judgment cannot be released until the 70,000 francs' cost of procedure are paid to the court. But, since the Union Meunière refuses to pay this, it is up to us to pay in advance, in turn to be reimbursed after the conclusion of the process. . . .

Mme. Mison, writing from the sanatorium at Ponteils, said that she would be able to borrow fifty thousand francs on the strength of the judgment, and wondered if it were possible for the association to lend her the balance of twenty thousand francs, which would be paid back immediately when she received the amount awarded her.

By Christmas time M. Carle and M. Delacquis were able to come forward with the needed money to receive official title to the judgment. By the end of 1958 it appeared that the last obstacle might be cleared for the reparation of at least one of the members of the fragile organization that had struggled so long in its fight.

Through December, and through January of the new year, M. Delacquis worried. There was no word whatever of progress in the case, and finally, as January was nearing its end, he wrote Maître Divol.

> On my advice and suggestion Madame Mison has collected together fifty thousand francs, and M. Carle and I have complemented it with a payment of twenty thousand francs of our own money, in the name of the association.
>
> I am astonished at not receiving any word and am disturbed by this silence, which seems to foreshadow another series of obstacles and evasions, of which we have had such an excessive amount.
>
> I have personally taken a heavy responsibility in persuading Mme. Mison to make this advance. I would not be able to admit that the affair is now buried, and that the judgment will remain simply a scrap of paper.
>
> I would be very thankful if you could put me up to date with the results of your progress, and count on the fact that you will be able to announce very soon a favorable outcome.

Once again M. Delacquis felt his hopes ebbing swiftly. It was the same feeling he had had during the years before, as the case dragged out interminably, the date for the trial postponed time and again. Further, his vision, his throat, and his vertigo were all becoming increasingly worse. His sense of responsibility gave him the deepest concern in that he had persuaded Mme. Mison to marshal a considerable amount of money on his recommendation, and now there seemed to be no assurance that she would even get that back—to say nothing of the award she had received from the court.

The attorneys, in the meanwhile, were not without their problems. They had contributed their time and even their money far beyond what the case would ever bring them in compensation. They were loathe to bill the association at all, knowing the straits in which it found itself. Yet so much of their other work had fallen behind that they were beginning to feel a serious pinch in the budget themselves. To compensate for it, they worked late at night and on weekends, but always with the problem that their staffs and overhead were continuing without adequate recompense.

For these reasons, M. Divol received with deep concern the news—even though it was expected—that the Union Meunière had appealed the decision of the Tribunal at Uzès, and was placing the case before the Court of Appeal in Nîmes. On receiving M. Delacquis's latest plea, he was faced with the problem of advising him of the latest move by the Union, and trying to explain another delay—this time one of the longest yet encountered.

> I acknowledge the receipt of your letter informing me of your disturbance at the thought of anticipating another series of obstacles in the progress of the procedure.
>
> I have indeed received from you the seventy thousand francs which will allow me to carry out the registration of the judgment, but I am not able to execute it at the moment since the Union Meunière has filed its appeal, and we must await the decision of the Court of Nîmes to call for (if of course the judgment is confirmed) the payment of the damages and interest allowed Mme. Mison, and for the others who have been disabled, after the medical experts have completed their mission. . . .
>
> Thus, I find that I must advise you that we must face a delay of a full year, or a year and a half, for the date to be set before the Court of Appeal.

Stunned by the news, and filled with embarrassment and sorrow at the thought of Mme. Mison, who was now faced with a large debt that she had no chance of repaying for over a year, at the least, he took the only action he could think of: To write directly to the Minister of Justice in Paris, and lodge the strongest protest he could. He realized, he was fully aware, that he was fighting windmills, that perhaps it would even do more harm than good. But to him, it was the only way he could keep his sanity.

> It will soon be eight years since the tranquil village of Pont-Saint-Esprit was stricken with the tragic affair that has been called by the press *le pain maudit*. . . .
>
> No one has been able to say exactly what the nature of the poison was, and who was responsible for this collective poisoning. . . .
>
> After delays and postponements without number, the Tribunal at Uzès has pronounced its judgment on April 24, 1958. The Union Meunière has been condemned. . . . Bravo! At last justice was done.
>
> Unfortunately, it has been necessary to change the tone. The brutal conclusion—here it is: It has been necessary for the victims to pay for the cost of the title of the judgment, since the Union Meunière refused to pay it. This is normal practice, apparently. Perhaps, yes, but it is a discouraging blow.
>
> But that is not all. I am informed now that the Union Meunière has filed an appeal, and that it is necessary to await the decision of the Court of Nîmes to call for the payment *if indeed the judgment is confirmed*. It will be necessary for the widow of M. Mison, whose husband was killed eight years ago, to wait a year to a year and a half more, merely to have the appeal brought before the court.
>
> We are only able to admit, *Monsieur le Ministre*, that those unfortunates who have suffered in their hearts and in their bodies as a result of the wrongs of the Union Meunière, have been repulsed as outcasts, as if someone were playing a tragic game with them. . . .
>
> If Justice has remained so slow and also so unjust, our country is shamed by it.
>
> I am certain, *Monsieur le Ministre*, that you will intervene in this affair, and that at length, those who await this justice will have it rendered to them before they are dead.

Maître Divol, understanding the sense of futility of his clients, but aware that M. Delacquis's appeal to the Minister of Justice would accomplish nothing, set about securing a lien on the property of M. Briand, and tried to calm his client's fury and frustration as best he could.

The major part of M. Delacquis's bitterness and anger arose from the feeling that he was responsible, because of the confidence so many people had placed in him. Time and again he had reassured the members, and in good faith, had indicated to them that positive action was certain to be forthcoming. He could not himself believe that the process would drag out so long over the years, and at every setback, had reassured himself that it would be the last.

Two years before the Pyrrhic victory at the Tribunal at Uzès, he had been ready to surrender. The trial at that moment was not even in sight. The obstacles had seemed too much for his fragile health to withstand. It was at this time, in the spring of 1956, that he met Wanda. He met her through her brother, a mason, who owned a small villa on the tiny, narrow Impasse Latour that was modest enough in price for M. Delacquis to consider buying and restoring to its seventeenth-century charm. Wanda fell in love with him at once. M. Delacquis, whose previous travels over the world had kept him a bachelor, was struck by her effervescence, her buoyancy, her constant cheerfulness, which brought him stamina when he needed it most.

He saw her often. Several times the thought crossed his mind that he would ask her to marry him. But each time he resisted the idea. With his sickness, he reasoned, he would be nothing but a burden, and in addition, at the age of fifty-seven, he was twenty years Wanda's senior.

It was Wanda who restored his courage and reignited his determination when he was ready to surrender. It was she who kept up his spirits in the most dolorous times, helped him on the long and exhausting bus trips to the eye specialist in Nîmes, cooked him lavish Italian meals at her brother's house, meals she had learned as a girl in her native Vintimiglia.

Just before the trial at Uzès, M. Delacquis blurted out what he had no intention of expressing.

He said: "If I were younger, I'd ask you to marry me."

She said: "I don't think there's so much difference."

Without hesitation, he said: "Let's get married."

They did, in June of 1959, and M. Delacquis later said that if it had not been for this joy, he would have lost all hope when the new obstacles arose after the long-awaited decision from the court, for the despair of the most needy among the association's members was contagious. It weighed him down with a sense of futility. Infused with new hope from the love and companionship of Wanda, he was able to set a new course and gain fresh resolve. "It is good," he said later, "for the heart to take over the mind."

He needed all the resolve he could muster when a new letter arrived from Mme. Mison, whose failing health was reflected in her weak and trembling handwriting.

"I must excuse myself for not yet being able to return the twenty thousand francs that you and M. Carle had the kindness to advance. My concern is for you, and what you must feel with year after year of delay. Yet happily, I do not lose hope. Again, my thanks for your patience."

M. Delacquis replied immediately, reassuring her about her concern in repaying the money. "It is necessary to arm ourselves with patience, and not lose courage," he said.

The patience of all, however, was strained again when M. Briand filed an appeal on his own part, bringing the case to a standstill on all fronts.

The legal bills, including the new appeals now being launched by M. Briand and the Union Meunière, had now mounted to astronomical amounts because of the complexity of the cases, and even though the lawyers had donated much of their time and money. Something had to be done about the bills, even if only a token payment, and M. Delacquis knew it. A summary of the out-of-pocket expenses of the lawyers alone was considerable. M. Delacquis, seeking funds from the members, had nowhere to turn. Everyone who could contribute had done so beyond the limit of their resources. Borrowing money was impossible. Mme. Mison, anxious to contribute her share, as the only case that specifically would receive immediate indemnification if the appeal were won, was unable to raise any more money beyond what she already had.

M. Delacquis now began to have new concern about the appeal, even if the victims were to win it: How could any medical examination be genuinely fair and effective nearly a decade after the people had been stricken?

Further, the appeal required the services of an additional *avoué* in Nîmes, adding further legal expense. In desperation, M. Delacquis wrote to a television show that dealt with controversial interviews, *Vous Êtes Formidable*, begging them to review the struggle in the hope that viewers might contribute money. But since the case was in the middle of litigation, the producers felt obliged to reject the idea.

Nerves were strained, tempers flared, some of the members revolted against the delays.

Another year passed, fruitlessly, painfully, slowly.

By February of 1960, however, nine years after the tragedy, the process began to crystallize again. The appeal was set for March 14, 1960. Representing the association would be Maître d'Everlange, of Nîmes, an associate of M. Divol.

"I hope sincerely," M. Delacquis wrote to Mme. Mison, "that this time your case will definitely be decided, and that you will be able to come into possession of the damages and interest that has been granted you."

The appeal was based on purely legal questions. No new question of fact would be introduced. Only the lawyers for all the clients concerned attended, and afterward, the three judges would study the pleas, and announce their decision at a later date.

They were reasonably prompt.

Again, the association clearly and without reserve won the case.

On April 25, Maître Bedos was able to write M. Delacquis: "As you have certainly learned by the press before receiving this letter, the court has today rendered its decision.

"It is, as far as we are concerned, the most complete success for which we could have wished."

The decision was exactly that. In addition to confirming the terms of the first trial, it provided that the cost of medical examinations would have to be provided for by M. Briand, who in turn would be guaranteed all his payments by the Union Meunière.

Mme. Mison's award was raised to 1,500,000 old francs, or approximately three thousand dollars.

Maître d'Everlange, confirming the letter from Maître Bedos, sent along the written opinion of the court. "You will see that, as far as our case is concerned, it is a very happy confirmation."

After nearly ten years of frustration, it was a total legal victory.

A victory that was to last for exactly one day.

FIFTEEN

In his preparations to notify the members of the association of the welcome news, M. Delacquis did not immediately open a second letter from his lawyers that arrived on his desk the next morning. He was extremely anxious to reassure Mme. Mison that her worry over the money she had borrowed was unnecessary, and to advise the other members that the cost of the medical research required by the decision would be covered by both the baker and the Union Meunière. This was a vitally important point because most of the members could not afford the costly process of detailed physical examinations, involving possible X rays, electroencephalogram tests, blood tests, and other laboratory analyses. Estimates from the board of medical men after the first court decision had, in fact, come to as high as twenty-five thousand old francs for each member, or nearly fifty dollars each, plus the cost of possible hospitalization for those who required lengthy examinations.

Preparing to dictate a letter of optimism to Mme. Mison, who still remained in the Sanatorium du Ponteil, he paused to open the lawyer's letter.

It was from Maître Bedos, and he stared at it in disbelief as he read it.

> A hearing, a little too rapid in the decision of the Court rendered yesterday morning, failed to reveal an important error concerning the case between M. Briand and the Union Meunière.
>
> The Court indicates, in effect, that the guaranty of the Union Meunière will only be accorded to M. Briand if it can be proved that the toxicity of the flour was caused by Panogen.
>
> Also, the Court calls upon the medical panel which has been appointed to appraise the consequences of the poisoning on the victims, to determine in their research *if* the poisonings actually are derived from the presence of Panogen.
>
> This reservation is important, because if, with the long passage of years, the experts are unable to confirm this, the recourse that M. Briand has against the Union Meunière becomes sterile and useless.
>
> This is why I am pleased, more than ever, that we placed our direct action against M. Briand, who remains the sole responsible person.

Whatever the case against M. Briand, the fact remained that his resources could not begin to cover the damages suffered by all the victims, to say nothing of the pilot case of Mme. Mison. Beyond that was the crucial point: Even the criminal investigation and the report of the toxicologists had not proved that the poisoning was caused by Panogen. The *Réquisitoire Definitif* had clearly stated: "In spite of all the research, the proof is not made that Panogen is at the base of the poisonings of Pont-Saint-Esprit." In addition, most of the medical men who had been most closely involved with the case would not even accept the theory of mercury as the cause.

Mercury—the base of the Panogen fungicide—had been found only in infinitesimal quantity in the viscera of only one victim, and none had been found in any of the samples of the flour or bread. How then could a physical examination, ten years after the event, indicate in any remote way the presence of mercury, to say nothing of proving that the mercury had arisen from the source of Panogen? Further, the symptoms revealed were almost totally foreign to those of mercury poisoning.

The theory that the actual source of the poisoning was a potent derivative of lysergic acid, derived spontaneously from ergot, was becoming more and more logical as more information of the deadly and mysterious new drug LSD-25 was being uncovered through the 1950's. But its properties at this time were still not widely enough known for any but the most informed to take seriously. As late as 1962 LSD was not recorded in the pharmacology curriculum. More data were emerging from the Swiss laboratories which confirmed the unique, concentrated power and impact of the drug—more data to indicate that the symptoms were strangely akin to the Pont-Saint-Esprit cases.

The compulsion to jump out of windows, frequent manifestation in Pont-Saint-Esprit, was to become a strong characteristic of LSD symptoms, including the conviction—expressed by M. Puche—that one could fly. (Many years later, Timothy Leary was to say: "Any idiot knows that you never take LSD above the ground floor.") The lack of sexual stimulation, per se, became evident in the LSD research, as well as the identical animal reactions and the constant reports of the distortion of time and space, the hallucinations of animals, the feeling that the walls and ceiling are closing in, the trembling, the profuse and chilled sweating, the weak pulse, the euphoria, the revulsion to tobacco, the insomnia, the compulsion to commit suicide, the strange desire to run naked (as Emile had done), and the compulsion to write endlessly (as M. Delacquis had done)—all of which had characterized the Pont-Saint-Esprit cases. Further, the frequent illusions of witnessing one's own funeral and the epilepsy-like seizures and convulsions beginning to show up in LSD tests, which at that time were confined to the laboratory or to selected doctors and volunteers, were definitely parallel to the Pont-Saint-Esprit syndromes. One victim of Pont-Saint-Esprit later gave birth to a child who was tragically deformed and retarded; this effect would later be noted in LSD victims. The hallmark of LSD and that of the Pont-Saint-Esprit tragedy were also identical: widely dilated pupils.

With LSD practically unknown to everyone during the 1950's, the strength of the drug was only slowly revealed to the layman. Colorless, tasteless, and odorless, two pea-sized tablets of LSD could hallucinate up to three thousand people. A billionth of a pound would be sufficient to cause hallucinations. Mercury has never shown such properties, in any form. Also, a natural and spontaneous form of lysergic-acid alkaloids creating LSD-type reactions was discovered in morning-glory seeds. The question as to what a concentrated, accidental overdose of lysergic acid could do was simply impossible to demonstrate without causing a tragedy as punishing as that of Pont-Saint-Esprit. "It is possible," said one doctor, "that LSD is simply the scientifically revealed cause of historical ergotism. The parallelism of the symptoms cannot be discounted or escaped, nor does it seem to be a coincidence."

M. Delacquis was no more aware of the growing similarity between what was being uncovered in the unbelievable theater of LSD research than were the police, the authorities, the lawyers, and the judges. Without direct observation of such unthinkable power, the new drug could only appear to be a mystical potion, as ephemeral as a condiment in a witch's brew. Intent on trying to bring an end to all the struggles over the years, M. Delacquis was concentrating on his reply to Mme. Mison, making it as cautiously optimistic as possible. He wrote the widow:

> In that which concerns your part of the court decision, the sum has now been set at 1,500,000 *anciens* francs, counting damages and interest. This must be paid to you by the Union Meunière, if it is recognized within the next two months that the poisoning was due to Panogen; or by M. Briand, in the contrary case.
>
> It remains for us to arm ourselves with patience one time more, and to await that which will at last end, this process which has appeared to us up until now so filled with obstacles of every nature.

Replying to him, Mme. Mison wrote: ". . . at last to be able to see this affair terminate, after nine years of patience. I count on you, M. Delacquis. . . . I pray nightly that there is some way I can repay you for all your pain and trouble. . . .

For M. Delacquis the pain and trouble continued. Confused by the many intricacies of the court decision, and attempting to clarify the status of the case in his own mind, so that he could explain it to the others, he wrote his lawyers:

> The full text of the court decision, although very interesting, does not clarify for me the things which concern:
>
> 1. The delay on which we must count to finally terminate the procedure in court.
>
> 2. The clear and definitive nature of the toxic agent.

3. The date when the damages for Madame Mison can definitely be expected.

In general the poisoned people poorly understand why it should be useful now, nine years after the poisonings, to know if they had been poisoned by Panogen, ergot, or by dead rats. . . .

In replying the next day to M. Delacquis's letter, Maître Bedos lost no time moving directly to the heart of the matter. Categorically, he answered the questions:

I am eager to respond to your letter of inquiry, but am afraid I must disappoint you one time more in that which concerns the practical solution to the problems.

1. An appeal to the Supreme Court is now foreseen, if not inevitable. Unfortunately this does not permit us to envisage a solution *before two more years.*

2. However, this does not hinder us from some recourse, first, in moving toward the work of the research in appraising the individual cases; and second, the execution of the condemnation against M. Briand in the case of Mme. Mison. . . .

He went on to explain that a lien was already held on the business funds and equipment of the baker, and that this could be exercised in the widow's favor. As far as the other victims were concerned, the amounts of their damages would be dependent on the results of their physical examinations.

Most important—and disheartening—he continued, was the fact that it now appeared that the Union Meunière had virtually disengaged itself from liability, in that even all the experts in France had not proved that the source of the poisoning was Panogen.

I am only able to join you and the victims in their discouragement and disgust at the evolution of the procedure, but I hope you will be able to understand that the fault does not lie in men, but in institutions.

Our magistrates are directed only to apply the laws that, conceived in the interest of the defense of individuals by the numerous guaranties they provide, end up by suffocating them.

To be certain of discovering the culpable, with all the rigors of proof required by the penal code and the scientists, the criminal investigation lasted for four years and ended up in a failure.

Then, to permit the defense to establish its rights, the civil courts have accomplished that of which you already are so aware.

But in carrying out the interest of the victims, there has not been any torpedoing of their cause, and often even, except in the early stages of the investigation, very much good faith and consideration.

Even more, and I will perhaps shock you, I will reveal to you that I even feared that most of the victims would be declared ineligible to reclaim damages, since there was some question that they could prove without any shadow of a doubt that they have bought their bread from M. Briand, public knowledge not being an acceptable substitute for proof of sale in each particular case. . . .

M. Delacquis passed along the dismal news to Mme. Mison, who remained the most urgent case of the many among the members, concluding his note by saying, "I vow that I am not going to accept defeat, and that I will follow this through as far as possible."

On August 29, 1960, the ninth anniversary of the *éclosion brutale* in the streets of Pont-Saint-Esprit, Mme. Mison wrote again from the sanatorium; her handwriting was now almost illegible. Four months had gone by since the Court of Appeal had granted her the new award—four months in which nothing had happened. She expressed her concern for the money she owed, and wondered whether all hope had now been completely lost.

M. Delacquis could give her no assurance, nor was there much to say on any count. Even by mid-November, the clerk of the court had not yet released the official copy of the court decision which would permit direct action in liquidating the assets of M. Briand; nor had the experts yet taken action to organize the plan to examine the victims. On November 12, 1960, he wrote to M. Bedos:

The days pass, and we see nothing accomplished. I persist, however, to believe that having accepted the task of being the spokesman for the victims of the poisonings of Pont-Saint-Esprit, I must continue my duty. Without searching further for the source of the shackles that make our lawsuit a parody of justice, I would like to

> know what I ought to say now to those who continually present me with questions. When and how will Mme. Mison receive the money which the court at Nîmes awarded her? The other victims—are they considered as victims or as puppets of no interest?
>
> Believe me, *cher maître*, that I do not seek to criticize your action. It simply seems inadmissable that nine years after the event the victims are unable to receive any compensation for their suffering and their expenses. . . .

But M. Bedos was suffering also. An important ambiguity in the court decision and an error by the clerk who prepared the final draft of the court decision combined to make it doubtful either that the case against M. Briand for the funds so desperately needed by Mme. Mison could be pressed until after a Supreme Court decision, years away, or that the victims themselves would not have to stand for the measurably high cost of the medical examination. Further than that, the new problems indicated that there was a possibility that if any of the victims refused to submit themselves to examination, they would be fined pro-rata for the amount of expense already engendered by the preparations for the research.

By the time Christmas arrived—and in spite of the ambiguities—the legal document of the judgment was released, and it appeared that the actual realization of the award to Mme. Mison might be forthcoming from M. Briand, who in turn would have to try to seek indemnification from the balking Union Meunière.

The new year—1961—began auspiciously. The official papers were ready to be served for the seizure of M. Briand's assets. The medical experts appointed by the court called for a meeting with the victims, even though the machinery would not be set in motion until spring.

The weight of the forthcoming appeal by the Union Meunière to the Supreme Court hung over everything, leaving doubts, uncertainties, and depression among the members of the association.

M. Bedos, writing to M. Delacquis to advise him of the estimates of the cost of the medical review, recognized the feelings that would be generated among the members. "I can foresee the reaction to these estimates already," he wrote, "but it is necessary to understand that the specialists must be compensated in some way for the complex work they will have to do, and that this cost is reimbursable if the ultimate end of the trial is achieved. . . .

He was not wrong in his estimate of the reaction of the victims. Each individual would have to pay the twenty-five thousand old francs from his own pocket for the examinations, plus up to twenty thousand more for the laboratory tests. For the serious cases requiring hospital internment for the tests, an additional levy of five thousand old francs would necessarily be imposed. In this manner, some individuals would have to pay as high as fifty thousand francs for a gamble which most likely could never result in their receiving indemnity.

Maître Bedos, faced with the obligation of passing this information on, knew that for all practical purposes the case of the victims could come to a dead halt right here. Even the more affluent of the members of the association could not afford this cost, to say nothing of the feeling predominant among all the group that nothing constructive could possibly be proved a decade after the event. But the attorney was faced with his own fight against the cumbersome institutions of the law, as well as the fact that he had to report to his clients the conditions that actually existed. If the appeal to the Supreme Court were not imminent, if the ambiguities could be quickly cleaned up, the picture would have been different. It was a case of winning in both instances before the court, only to find his clients faced with putting out more money in order to gain their rights, which might eventually go up in the smoke created by a Supreme Court decision against it.

M. Delacquis, however, took up the fight again. He doggedly prepared a notice concerning the cost of the projected examinations, and waited for the response from the members.

It was not long in coming. And the response was what both he and Maître Bedos had expected.

After years of attrition, the victims could simply not raise the money.

Further, they were swamped in a feeling of defeat and hopelessness in the face of the engines of justice which constantly sputtered and died all through the decade. M. Delacquis wrote in despair to Maître Bedos:

The tests by the medical experts come, in effect, at so late a time that it seems to all here to be one measure more to make us give up and recoil from it. After nearly ten years the medical dossiers and the professors charged with the research will scarcely be able to change what exists now. We do not refuse, however, to appear before this medical commission. But the cost that would be imposed on us is too great for our purse. It is not, therefore, an act of ours to perform an act of abandonment. If we are given the financial means, we will appear. We still do not understand why the cost should be ours, rather than that of those who are responsible.

You see, Maître, that I am brokenhearted to arrive at this conclusion, but I believe that we now find ourselves at a total impasse. Nevertheless, I turn to you, our defender, and ask you: Is there nothing more to be done? What do we do after having buried our dead, buried our illusions and hopes?

If the terms that I employ give you the impression that I am unjust, I pray you to forgive me, you see only the manifestation of a shocked consciousness. . . .

The reaction to the bad turn events had taken since the ostensible victory in the courtroom hung like a pall over the village.

"Ten years after," said one victim, "what will the experts be able to discover?"

"My husband and my daughter have both been terribly sick," said another, "but slowly they have been regaining their health. Now, they are almost cured. What good would any new examination do?"

"How can we raise twenty-five thousand francs, each of us?" said a third. "And even if we could, and we were judged disabled, suppose then they cannot prove that we have been poisoned by Panogen? We have lost money we would have to borrow, and we would have no further help from anyone."

Events moved swiftly through the rest of 1961. The pattern of hope and failure continued in almost predictable waves.

Five months after the Court of Appeal had rendered its decision, the Association of Bakers came to the support of M. Briand, and enabled him to pay the damages to Mme. Mison, who at last was able to pay off her accumulated debts.

Three months later, she died.

The ambiguity concerning the cost of the medical examinations was at last clarified. And as another new year began, the beginning of the physical examinations was in sight.

On January 27, 1962, M. Delacquis prepared an official announcement for the members of the association and stamped it with the rubber stamp bearing the association's name—now worn and crumbled from the voluminous correspondence over the decade.

> The victims who desire to present themselves to the experts at Montpellier are asked to register at my office at the Cooperative of Cereals before February 10, 1962.
>
> The secretary reminds those who are interested that the cost of the examinations will not be charged to the members, but those who refuse the examination will risk being condemned to pay the cost accrued.

Not one member of the association registered for the process.

Three years later, on January 21, 1965, the first Civil Chamber of the Supreme Court at Paris rejected the appeal by the Union Meunière, and confirmed the decision of the Court of Appeal at Nîmes.

The association had won its case again, in the highest court of the land.

M. Delacquis, in the garden of his tiny villa on Impasse Latour, read the news in the paper with his right eye, his left almost completely blind. He passed the paper across to Wanda, who looked at it, then turned away from him. She was crying.

In the Grande Rue, in the *tabacs* and cafés along the Boulevard Gambetta the news was passed from villager to villager, almost without comment. There were abrupt nods, shrugs, or a sad, slow shaking of the head. There were sad and terrifying memories evoked; there were some few curt, gruff comments, all of them bitter, ironic, or full of apathetic resignation.

There were no cries for action, no smiles of triumph. There was only the desire to forget.

Wanda Delacquis rose from her garden chair, still unable to look at her husband. She entered the thick stone doorway of the house, crossed the dining room to a small cabinet, took out the dusty envelopes holding the files of the association. Carefully she untied the cord that held them together, then placed the newspaper inside it, next to a bank statement marked *Closed.*

M. Delacquis, walking shakily from the garden, stood in the doorway and watched her as she tied the cord around the big envelope, then placed it back in the cabinet. The rubber stamp had fallen out on the floor, and she bent down, picked it up, dropped it far back into the cabinet. M. Delacquis shuffled toward her, holding on to the dining room table for support. There were tears in his eyes, too. He placed his trembling hands tenderly on her shoulders and kissed her on the forehead.

On the hill above Pont-Saint-Esprit, the statue of the Virgin looked out across the plains of the Rhône Valley. Wisps of smoke were punctuating the fields where the dried vines from the vintage year were burning to clear the vineyards for the coming year. The statue of Mary, imperturbable, unchanged, held out both her arms in the attitude of grace. The broken arm had long since been repaired, and many hundreds of the faithful had made pilgrimages since 1951 to the high tower on which she stood.

From her vantage point, the mosaic of the tile rooftops of Pont-Saint-Esprit looked like an etching of a sleepy town in the Middle Ages. Under the roofs there were those who would never know peace or health again, and those who were thankful that they had escaped the ravages of a scourge that would forever, perhaps, remain a mystery.

EPILOGUE

I READ of the case of the "accursed bread" seventeen years ago, in a small news item in *The New York Times,* datelined Paris, August 28, 1951. The headline: THREE DIE, MANY STRICKEN BY MADNESS FROM POISON IN BREAD IN FRANCE, was singularly arresting. It seemed unbelievable in the age of scientific explosion that a rare disease of the Middle Ages could suddenly reappear. The last French epidemic of historical ergotism had been reported in Burgundy, north of the Pont-Saint-Esprit region in 1816.

But in 1951 France was having one of its wettest summers. Ergot was known to proliferate under wet, humid conditions. Ergot forms on patches of rye. One field may be seriously ridden with the parasitic growth, but the next patch may be in another field, several kilometers away. The harmful concentrations of ergot are most likely to survive in a small mill, where only small quantities of grain are milled at any one time. If the mill is processing grain from a single farmer, most of the grain can be totally free of ergot while portions of it can contain a high concentration.

From the *Times* article it was obvious that here was a medical mystery story of fascinating interest and intense drama. I clipped out the story, put it in my overstuffed idea file, and promptly forgot about it.

It was not until 1957, six years later, that the news item came back to mind again. I was at that time writing a regular column for the *Saturday Review,* and had just completed a piece on the work of Dr. R. B. Rhine and Dr. Karl Osis in the field of parapsychology. Dr. Rhine was kind enough to write from Duke University to tell me that the column was one of the more lucid pieces on the subject he had read, and that he hoped that I would follow up with others to clarify the scientific research being done in the subject.

Several months later I received a call from Dr. Osis, who asked me if I would be interested in exploring a new and revolutionary step in the probing of the deepest workings of the human mind. We arranged for an appointment in his office on 57th Street in New York.

At the meeting Dr. Osis explained that the research in a Swiss laboratory had accidentally uncovered a new drug, derived from ergot, which had created strange and unpredictable reactions on those volunteers who had tried it. Since it was among the most powerful drugs yet discovered, only infinitely small quantities were used in the experiments. At this time small samples of the drug were being circulated to serious and competent researchers in order to explore the consciousness-expanding qualities of the drug. The general public knew nothing about its properties, or for the most part, that it even existed. No journalists had yet been invited to write about it, and I would be the first to have the information, if I wished it.

Beyond that, it would be possible, if I so desired, to take the drug in the presence of a competent physician and psychologist, under carefully controlled conditions, and to report my own personal reaction in complete detail.

Dr. Osis explained that it would involve an entire day in the office, beginning at nine o'clock in the morning, and extending straight through until evening. The dosage would be administered orally, and the doctor and psychologist would be in attendance throughout the day. He warned, however, that sometimes the drug could create extremely adverse reactions. If this turned out to be the case, the physician would be ready at any time to take countermeasures in the form of tranquillizers. Dr. Osis also made it a point to emphasize that I should not consider the idea if I were undergoing any particular period of strain at the time. This condition would almost certainly engender the adverse reactions, and the experiment would be useless in exploring the consciousness-expanding qualities of the drug.

At this particular time I had just completed a new play, which was ready to go into rehearsal for its pre-Broadway tour. I was in the middle of last minute rewrites, always a painful and chaotic period of stress. I explained to Dr. Osis that I had better think it over before committing myself, but that I appreciated very much the chance for a scoop on what seemed to be a most unusual story.

That evening I gave the idea serious consideration. I always enjoyed writing stories that, if carefully documented and conservatively written, would strike out into new and unexplored fields. Whatever this new drug was, it sounded incredible. The chance to be the first journalist to document the story was even more tempting. But with my play on the eve of rehearsal, with casting problems and endless conferences with Alfred Drake, the director, with the agony of the pre-Broadway tour through New Haven, Boston, and Philadelphia staring me in the face, I felt that I would regretfully have to decline the invitation.

I called Dr. Osis the next morning, thanked him profusely for the chance of a scoop. Then I turned back to working on the script of the play. My mind kept wandering back to the story however, and I suddenly remembered the *Times* clipping from eight years before about the little village on the banks of the Rhône. Wasn't ergot at the base of the poisonings? Wasn't ergot also the base of this new and powerful drug Dr. Osis had talked to me about?

I dug out the *Times* clipping, now beginning to yellow in the overstuffed folder. Yes, it was ergot that had apparently caused nearly three hundred people in the village to go madly insane, some of them jumping out of windows, others into the Rhône, in what must have been a scene directly out of Dante's *Inferno*. If ergot were related to the new drug, which it of course was, there was an obvious danger in any accidental overdose.

I was glad, in one way, that I had turned the experiment down. But I made a mental note that it would be extremely interesting to investigate the story of Pont-Saint-Esprit some day, to see if by any chance there were some relationship between the new drug just beginning to emerge into active experimentation, and the strange psychogenic drama that took place in Pont-Saint-Esprit.

It was not until nearly eight years later that the idea returned to me again. Partly because LSD-25 had grown into a monstrous problem, and partly because the Pont-Saint-Esprit drama lingered in my mind as a classic tragedy and an absorbing medical mystery story, I decided that I would go to France and investigate the story first hand. I had just completed two books, *Incident at Exeter*, and *The Interrupted Journey*, each of which was gratifyingly successful, and which dealt with the strange, relatively unexplored subject of Unidentified Flying Objects, in what I hoped was a thoroughly responsible style of journalism. I could afford, I felt, to take the risk of a trip to France, even if it turned out to be a wild goose chase.

I was fortunate enough to have a friend, Larry Michel, whose mother was one of the senior editors of the large-circulation newspaper *France-Soir*, and who kindly offered to give me any assistance I needed in exploring the story, which was now over fifteen years old. My French was rusty, but I took a crash course at a Berlitz language school, which gave me enough shaky confidence to begin the research.

I arrived in the bitter cold Paris of January, 1967, and thanks to Mme. Yvonne Michel, literally buried myself in the dusty morgue of the *France-Soir* archives.

The file on the Pont-Saint-Esprit case of *le pain maudit* was voluminous. Every newspaper in France had carried major stories on it, at great length. The story began with a small clipping datelined August 22, 1951, and continued through the years to January 21, 1965, when the Supreme Court decision was announced, in another Pyrrhic victory for the victims.

But, for the first time, I was startled to find that the police and the courts no longer considered that historical ergotism was the cause. Instead, the mercurial fungicide theory had been accepted, and had been the basis for all the legal action which had lingered on through the years.

At first I was disappointed. But after studying the clippings for nearly seven days, eight or nine hours a day, and laboriously translating them, I felt that the story was just as fascinating whether ergot poisoning was involved or not. The tragedy of the villagers in the town emerged from the pages of the dusty clippings vividly. It was a classic story that should be told, I was convinced, a modern medical detective story of absorbing interest both in and out of France.

With profuse thanks for her help I said good-bye to Mme. Michel, and drove down to the Midi.

The problems of exploring the story were of course obvious. Aside from the language barrier, I had been warned that the villagers of Provence and Languedoc were cold, distant, and uncommunicative with strangers. While they had a spirit and *joie de vivre* which was often lacking in the Parisian, it would take an outsider a very long time to crack the crust.

Beyond that, it was obvious that the story of the "accursed bread" was a sensitive one. It was still basically unsolved, and those who had lost loved ones or whose friends and relatives had been permanently disabled or crippled by the disease would be loathe to talk to a stranger about it, especially with the language barrier. After two weeks in Berlitz and a week in Paris I was hardly a master of the French language. In a town as small as Pont-Saint-Esprit, I would only be in the village ten minutes before I would be spotted as a stranger, stared at curiously, and rejected as a snooper. Further, the signs scrawled on deserted barns, stone bridges, and rocks along the highway driving south were not very encouraging: U.S. ASSASSINS . . . U.S.A. N'A PAS RAISON . . . YANKEE MEURTRIER . . . SAUVONS VIET NAM . . .

I decided that in order to discover the feeling of the town, and to try to get to know some of the people in a calm and unstrained atmosphere, I would have to practice a mild, benevolent deception. I knew no one whatever in the village, and had heard that it was almost certain that no one there could speak English. With my stumbling French it would be impossible to begin any depth-interviewing without getting to know some of the people well enough to beg their indulgence. I counted heavily on the tape recorder, so that I could listen and relisten to the interviews in French, and pick up the phrases I would lose in the thick Provençal and Languedoc accents of the Midi.

I decided at the outset not to stay in Pont-Saint-Esprit itself until I had a chance to get to know something about the town and the attitude of the people. The benevolent deception was to be the guise that I was going to write a series of magazine articles on the south of France, especially a story about the bridges over the Rhône, which would include those of Avignon and Pont-Saint-Esprit. I knew that I would want historical background about the town anyway, and by doing this research first, I gradually could move into the story of the "accursed bread" after I had gained a better capacity to deal with the subtleties of the southern French accent.

I stayed in Avignon, some forty kilometers away, and began several days of library research about the region and its history.

It was fascinating. The historical soil was so rich that it began to dim my interest in the main story. Further, it was a comfortable way of avoiding that first critical assault on the village, where a false move on my part could conceivably seal the lips of the villagers forever.

As I worked in the library of the Musée Calvet, in the imposing shadow of the Palais des Papes, I felt drawn into the region and its history with such power that I could not bring myself to break away from the fascinating volumes of the past, and move into the journalistic reality of the present. I was constantly plagued with fears and doubts. Whom would I speak to first in the village? How could I approach them diplomatically? Could I make myself well enough understood? Would they maintain the reticence toward strangers that characterized the small villages of France? Would they penetrate the innocent guise I had created about the bridges over the Rhône? I had been warned that the Frenchman of the Midi is instinctively shrewd and smart; that he could penetrate any disguise in a matter of moments. None of this was comforting, because I was not a good liar in English, to say nothing of French.

In a rented Peugeot, and trying to look as inconspicuous as possible, I drove from Avignon up the Rhône, and across the multiarched bridge of Pont-Saint-Esprit. On the river bank, the ancient *église* dominated the irregular, tiny houses clustered around it, mothering them as if they were an enormous litter it was trying to shield from the past ravages of the town's turbulent history. Along the Boulevard Gambetta the plane trees were stark and naked, reaching their scrawny branches toward the sky as if in supplication. The mistral was whipping through the streets bitterly, whistling through the branches, stirring up gusts of dust and leaves. Only a few villagers were braving it, bending down head forward to counterbalance its unrelenting force.

I parked the car in the Allées Frédéric Mistral—named for the poet of course, not the wind—and set out on foot to find the hat-and-sporting-goods shop of M. Boudenne. He was the local reporter for several French newspapers and had been recommended by a journalist in Avignon as the person who would be knowledgeable in the ways and mores of the town and region, even though he did not speak English.

I found him in the tiny office in the back of his sporting goods shop, buried under boxes of tennis shoes, *boules* sets, sunglasses, soccer balls, and inflatable kayaks. The shop was chilly and drafty, and little defense against the gusty mistral. He was wearing, as his own personal armor against it, a top coat and a slouch felt hat. Chubby and congenial, he greeted me cordially as I squeezed into the office.

"*Je suis un journaliste américain,*" I stumbled out, "*et j'écris une histoire concernant les ponts sur le Rhône, peut-être pour un magazine aux États-Unis.*"

"*Ah bon,*" he said. "*L'histoire du pont ici est très intéressante. Alors, est-ce possible que je vous aide?*"

I was surprised and delighted with his friendliness, and before long we were calling each other *mon cher confrère*, a development that dissolved many of my fears.

M. Boudenne was not only congenial, he was well informed. Since I was ostensibly only interested in the history of the town and the ancient bridge, he outlined for me a great deal of source material available in the archives of the town hall, and insisted on personally taking me across the Boulevard Gambetta to the Hôtel de Ville to introduce me to the town official who handled the small library and the ancient records of the village. I set up an appointment for the next day, since the archives were being closed for the afternoon.

On the way back across the street, I noticed a gendarme writing out a ticket for my car, which I soon was to discover was parked in an area labeled *Disque Obligatoire*, in which all cars had to display a disc available at any gas station, which could be rotated to show the time at which the car was parked. M. Boudenne gently chastised the officer for giving a ticket to "*un journaliste américain,*" and insisted on taking me back across the street to the police station, where he introduced me to the desk officer, and arranged to have my ticket canceled. I insisted that I was quite willing to pay the fine, but neither M. Boudenne nor the desk officer would hear of it.

The first day in Pont-Saint-Esprit could not have begun better.

The next morning, after spending the night in Avignon, I returned to thank M. Boudenne for his helpfulness, prior to going to the Hôtel de Ville for local historical research. The story of the bridges sounded so interesting that I felt I might actually do it.

I had no sooner entered the shop, when the congenial M. Boudenne came out of his office looking as if he were a cat who had swallowed a bird.

"Ah, monsieur," he said, shaking his head from side to side. "You did not tell me the truth yesterday! Shame on you."

I was startled by his change of attitude, and immediately thought of the comments I had heard in Paris about the perspicacity of the villagers in the Midi.

"Pardon?" I said, trying to look as innocent as possible.

He shook his head again, sadly, wistfully, as if I had lied and taken advantage of his good offices. Of course, I had. And I was ready to take my punishment and apologize to him, and to explain that I knew of no other way to go about the clumsy problem of entering a town cold turkey with such a poor command of the language.

"*Vous avez raison,*" I said, still wondering how he had penetrated my guise so quickly and easily. "You are absolutely right. I apologize."

"Why did you not come right out and tell me the real story you are here to investigate?" he said.

I stumbled around awkwardly, trying to find the right French words to express the subtleties of my apprehension and concern.

"So you came here to write the story of the Unidentified Flying Objects which have been reported," he said. "I did not know that they had received such international attention. But obviously they have."

I was completely stunned. I had said nothing about the subject of UFO's—or *soucoupes volantes* as they are called in France. I had not even hinted at the subject, which was one I wanted to avoid getting further involved in, after the two books on it. I did not want to get typed as a writer specializing in any particular subject. But his new assumption, of course, provided me with a far better "cover," until I got used to the atmosphere of the town, than the apocryphal story of the bridges over the Rhône. I fell right into the accusation gladly.

"Yes," I said. "You have uncovered my benevolent guise with impossible speed. I apologize profusely."

M. Boudenne smiled and shook my hand. "No need to apologize at all," he said. "We all practice little deceits. I have done so many times. But tell me—what are these strange objects? Six months ago, some of our finest citizens, including the mayor of Saint-Paulet-de-Caissons, reported seeing them not more than a meter above the ground."

"First you've got to tell me," I said, "just how you uncovered my decoy so quickly."

M. Boudenne went on to explain that my name had sounded vaguely familiar, and that he recalled having seen it in the French periodical *L'Express,* which was a big circulation weekly news magazine. Some weeks before I had arrived in France, this publication had run a long, two-part condensation of *Incident at Exeter,* the story of the amazing case of the Exeter, New Hampshire, police who were approached by an enormous UFO not more than one hundred feet above their heads, and had dropped to the ground in order to avoid it hitting them. Their case had proved out to such a degree that the U.S. Air Force had written to apologize to them for discounting the story at the beginning.

In the village of Pont-Saint-Esprit, I was to learn of a series of almost exactly the same nature as those of Exeter. Although the subject was digressionary in my present situation, I felt that it would be an excellent way to get to know the village before beginning the research on the story of the "accursed bread."

As a result, I did not hesitate to go along with M. Boudenne's assumption that I was in Pont-Saint-Esprit to explore the UFO story.

As it turned out, it was dramatic and convincing in itself, and an extremely tempting story to write as a magazine article. Three persons, all of them well regarded in the community, had viewed the object at different times. One farmer observed it as it swung down silently from the sky, and hovered not more than five or six feet above his field, then shot off in the sky at an incredible speed. The parallel to the Exeter sightings, thousands of miles away, was startling. Along with Robert James, the correspondent in Pont-Saint-Esprit for *Le Midi Libre,* I went out to Saint-Paulet-des-Peyrolas, interviewed the farmer involved, and the mayor of the village. The story checked out very well. But I was not specifically interested in writing it at the moment, and I went through the motions of the interviews wishing I could figure a way to transfer the subject matter to *le pain maudit* gracefully.

Within days my picture had appeared in all the newspapers of southern France in regard to the UFO story, and O.R.T.F., the national television network of France, sent an eight-man documentary film crew to the village to interview me on the parallelisms between the Pont-Saint-Esprit UFO sightings and those of Exeter. It was a good story, and I was still tempted to write it. And it enabled me to be in the town without arousing too much attention to the main story. After the newspaper and television publicity, I became somewhat of a pseudocelebrity in the town, which was helpful in getting to know the tradesmen, the bartenders, and the villagers more quickly.

The publicity also brought me in touch with the Eynards, the husband and wife who were both practicing dentists, and whose gracious hospitality, intelligence, and historical knowledge of the village were invaluable in learning about the region.

Through their help, and that of M. Boudenne, I gradually began to learn about the hidden wells and springs of the story of the "accursed bread." I met some of the victims, crippled and disabled by the poisoning, barely holding on to life in many cases. I heard their stories, most of which were heartbreaking. I learned of the conflict between the medical doctors and the toxicologists, of how the case still remained a deep and seemingly impenetrable mystery.

After beginning to learn some of the details behind the headlines, it was obvious that I could not conceive of writing the book without in some way sharing with the victims who had gone through a decade and a half of litigation without any indemnification in spite of their victories in three different courts, all the way up to the Supreme Court. I arranged to share a measurable portion of the royalties with the now-inactive Association for the Defense of the Victims of the Poisoning by the Bread of Pont-Saint-Esprit.

As the research began in earnest, and after confessing that the story of the bread was now my major objective, I learned that there were many ambiguities about the case, that the general feeling persisted that the entire case was squashed by the government of that time in order to avoid the possibility of having to pay out the millions of francs the indemnification would total.

I was also lucky to find a British journalist from Cannes, Ted Clark, who spoke French fluently, and who came up to Pont-Saint-Esprit, Nîmes, and Montpellier with me on several occasions to help out in the research. Even with the taped interviews I had done, I still had trouble translating their subtleties, and Clark and I spent long hours trying to unravel them. At times it seemed so difficult to continue with the placer-mining for the details of the story, that I was ready to toss the whole idea aside and forget about it. Clark would pour a double Scotch and keep me going on these occasions, which were not infrequent.

Above all, however, I came to love the village and the people in it wholeheartedly. After the superficial shell of resistance to strangers was cracked open, there could not be a more hospitable person than the Provençal. Along with his fatalistic acceptance of tragedy, was a resilient fountain of joy and wit which continually bubbled to the surface, leavening the moments of sadness as they were recalled.

Grande Rue, I was told, had hardly changed since that fateful day when the clients of M. Briand filed into his bake shop to buy their long loaves of bread, or the round, dome-shaped *pain de campagne*. There was one significent change, however: The bake shop of M. Briand was no longer there. Instead, it has become his insurance office, where he acts as a broker for several companies. He sits at his desk behind a steel counter in his office, surrounded by metal files, with the store window painted to make it opaque. He is a tall, pale man, with a huge frame and a sadness in his lined face that seems to reflect the scars of the terrible events that took place so long ago. He is not averse to talking about the tragedy if the listener is attentive and interested. He feels above all that he himself is as much, if not more, of a victim than any of the others. "If I had been a chemist," he said to me, "I might have been able to stop the terrible thing before it happened. But I'm not a chemist, and I had to depend on the quality controlled by the Union Meunière."

He is a deeply religious man, and it is his faith, some say, that kept him going since he had to close his bakery after thirty years, and begin over again with a new career. He has made a pilgrimage to Lourdes with his family to gain new faith and strength in the face of what he has had to bear.

M. and Mme. Testevin still run their vineyards with infinite love and care. Both show the same paleness that most of the victims seem to have inherited. M. Testevin, with a shy and wistful smile, does not like to think about his long days and nights on his bed. Mme. Testevin, now in her seventies, still manages La Villette with a happy acceptance of her chores and a thousand memories of her twenty days in purgatory. The former Bouvier house sits on the hill overlooking Pont-Saint-Esprit in quiet dignity. "If Jackie Kennedy would like to visit it," Mme. Testevin said, "we'd love to have her."

Emile is the only other one of the group who lived in the house during the time of crisis who still remains there today. In spite of his bent frame and his sharp and vivid memories of the nightmares, his smile is warm and contagious. He works long hours in the vineyards, even when his strength fades during those times when the symptoms of the poisoning return. He is back now in his little room above the stable wing, but joins the family for meals and wine and conversation in the evening.

Down the road less than a kilometer, the Rigaud sisters live in their spotlessly clean Provençal *mas*, recalling with a sense of horror the scenes that greeted them each day as they came to the aid of Mme. Testevin. One of their worst fears had been those times when M. Delacquis, and sometimes M. Testevin and Emile, had wanted to throw themselves out of a window. They could face almost anything but that with reasonable calm.

The Eynards, who escaped the ravages of the bread by accident, have a bustling dental practice on the Boulevard Gambetta, and a new villa on a hill on the road to Carsan. From their terrace the view of the Rhône Valley and Mont Ventoux in the distance is breathtaking. In spite of long hours in their office, they take time off to ski, camp, and foster the historical association of the village, which is fighting to preserve the Citadel, the underground cathedral, and other landmarks of medieval times that are crumbling from lack of funds to keep them in repair.

They took me through the tiny streets of the village to see Mme. Charpail, who is recovered now, except for occasional spells of dizziness, and M. Sauvet, now a widower, who is able to look back on his acrobatic escapades with a gentle sense of humor. "I was always so afraid of heights," he says, "and why I was compelled to go up on that bridge, I will never know."

M. Boudenne, when I first mentioned the story of the "accursed bread," characteristically shook his hand as if he had touched a hot stove. He said it was a story that no village in the world had ever gone through. He and his wife were only slightly affected by the disease, and they continue to laugh about how Mme. Boudenne wanted to punch him as hard as she could. Their hospitality was warm and generous. When I left Pont-Saint-Esprit, M. Boudenne was sitting in the sun on a camp chair, glancing through a newspaper in front of his shop, with the printed legend on the awning above him reading TOUT POUR LE SPORT.

Mme. Moulin lives alone on the isolated *domaine* outside of Pont-Saint-Esprit, although her helper and family live nearby. Having lost both her husband and son she faces a life of loneliness, but does so courageously and calmly. "*C'était penible!*" is the way she sums up the time of the crisis, though words could never express what she went through.

The *alimentation* shop of M. Carle is clean, prosperous, and busy. M. Carle and his family live above it, in spacious and attractive quarters, philosophically accepting the abortive struggle of the association, into which he put so much time, and so much of his own money. But Marie-Joseph has fully recovered, a vital and attractive girl who is studying to be a dietician.

Mlle. Wullschleger still comes to visit M. and Mme. Delacquis, having retired as secretary for the Coopérative des Céréales. She will say that there has never been a better boss than hers, and she helps Mme. Delacquis whenever he suffers a frequent relapse.

M. Delacquis, blind in one eye, and walking with great difficulty, can hardly speak above a whisper. But his mind remains strong and alert, and his wife is attentive and cheerful. I spent long hours in the little villa of M. Delacquis on the Impasse Latour. In a voice barely audible he responded to his wife Wanda, who in turn interpreted the answers in simple French for me. Around his dining room hang several of his oils, delicate and carefully wrought landscapes of subdued tones and appealing warmth. His bitterness concerning the long struggle over the years has given way to acceptance, though occasionally anger will flair up as he recalls the scenes of the past. He has been retired now from his work at the cooperative for several years.

Dr. Gabbai and Dr. Vieu continue their daily rounds in the village, settled down now to the common ailments of the ordinary community. There is no concern about a recurrence, for there is no better bread anywhere in France now than in Pont-Saint-Esprit. The bakeries are as spotless as laboratories. Tonsils, chickenpox, measles, flu, bronchitis, and all the other mundane afflictions occupy the doctors now, along with the births and deaths that march through the years everywhere. Dr. Channac is no longer living.

While I did not discuss any personal symptoms of the victims with any of the doctors, the villagers themselves advanced detailed information, which could be checked with the voluminous, impersonal medical journal reports on the outbreak, thus enabling me to piece together a mosaic which would give a valid picture of the scenes in the town during the time of crisis. In order to do this, a certain amount of extrapolation was necessary, but all of it was kept within the confines of the data available, which was enough to fill several cardboard cartons with research material. The transcriptions of the taped interviews themselves covered scores of pages from which much of the story was pieced together. In some cases, the recall of one witness differed from that of another, and a certain amount of guesswork was necessary to choose the most logical. Most important, I tried to capture accurately the mood and atmosphere of the village as it fought against one of the strangest phantoms in history.

This fight against phantoms was one of the most characteristic features of the entire story. It was for this reason that there were no real villains in the *coup de théâtre,* except perhaps fate.

Historical ergotism had not been experienced to any extent for so many epochs that no one could be expected to know of its dangers, or how to avoid it if they did. The farmers, the millers, the bakers involved in both the crucial outbreak in Pont-Saint-Esprit, and in the satellite outbreaks in the surrounding villages, were as puzzled, confused, and disturbed as those who tried to unravel the infinitely complex threads of the story. The major crux of the problem lay in quality control, and this, by prima-facie evidence, was simply not adequately provided for by the distribution system.

Near the end of my interviews and research I was able to interview both Dr. Giraud and Dr. Latour in Montpellier. Both of these distinguished men had prepared the bulk of the reports for the French Academy of Medicine, after having spent long days and nights in Pont-Saint-Esprit attempting to trace the cause of the poisonings, and to aid the overworked doctors in the village.

It was at this time that I was surprised to learn that the findings of the doctors involved were opposed to those of the toxicologists. The symptoms were not those of mercury poisoning, but were clearly those of historical ergotism. It had seemed that once the police found traces of mercury, they stopped there and looked no further.

This was a major, critical point, and affected the entire course of the painful and laborious civil cases. Mercury affects mainly the liver and the kidneys, and these organs were not significantly damaged in the Pont-Saint-Esprit cases. On the other hand, the symptoms, both psychogenic and cardiovascular, were exactly those of historical ergotism. Mercury salts are used in all of agriculture as pesticides and fungicides, and this could easily lead to the discovery of traces of mercury, in nonlethal and nontoxic doses.

The crux of the matter seemed to lie in the fact that historical ergotism itself had never been explained. Further, the alkaloids released by the fermentation of ergot deteriorate much faster than those of mercury. The laboratory examination of the Pont-Saint-Esprit victims came at a time too late to detect any significant amount of ergot alkaloids, even if they had been present. LSD enters the blood in ten minutes and starts a mysterious chain reaction that continues on its own momentum after the acid has disappeared. Practically no evidence of the drug is found in either the urine or exhaled breath, to say nothing of the body organs.

But there were traces of ergot alkaloids discovered in far more samples than contained mercury. The problem was that hardly anyone outside of the Swiss laboratories knew anything about the then-rare and strange form of ergot which was so dramatically powerful and concentrated that it was hard to conceive.

Dr. Giraud was kind enough to give me the full medical reports prepared for the Academy, and I took them back to my hotel in Nîmes to study. I had already prepared the basic outline for the book, which would lead naturally from the ergot theory, and conclude with the mercury theory. But it was then that I discovered the section in the report on LSD-25.

Suddenly the story had twisted back to the premise that had stirred my interest.

Whatever is the true answer to the mystery will probably never be known. The fact remains that the doctors and the toxicologists remain locked in an impasse.

But as one doctor expressed his opinion: "There is one and only one cause of the tragedy: Some form of ergot, and that form has logically got to be akin to LSD."

INDEX

INDEX

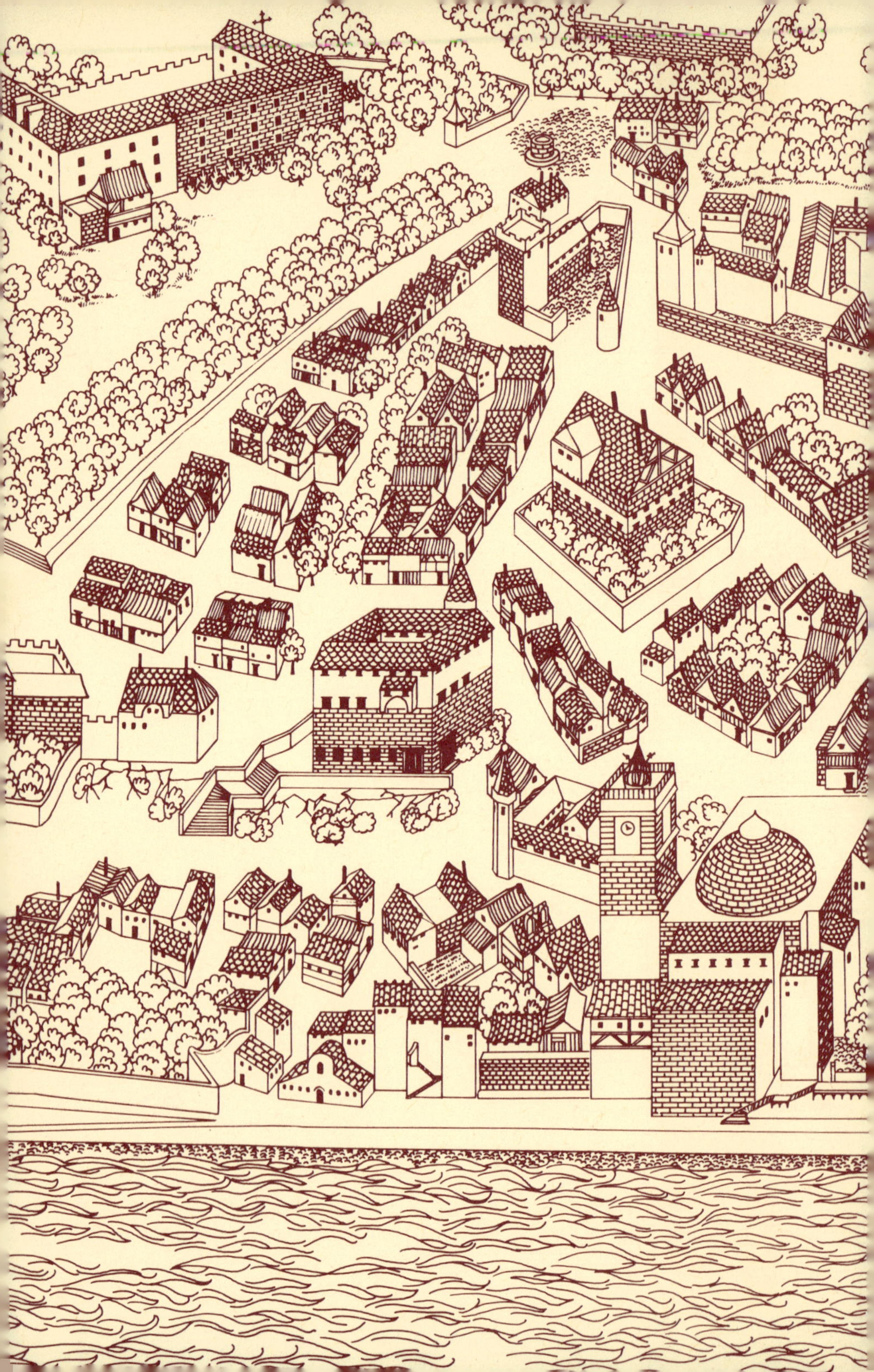